THE
DASH
DIET
Weight Loss
Solution

THE

DASH DIET

Weight Loss Solution

**2 WEEKS TO DROP POUNDS,
BOOST METABOLISM,
AND GET HEALTHY**

Marla Heller, MS, RD

GRAND CENTRAL
PUBLISHING

NEW YORK   BOSTON

Grand Central Publishing
Hachette Book Group
1290 Avenue of the Americas, New York, NY 10104
grandcentralpublishing.com
twitter.com/grandcentralpub

Printed in the United States of America

LSC-C

First trade paperback edition: December 2019

10 9 8 7 6 5 4 3 2 1

Grand Central Publishing is a division of Hachette Book Group, Inc. The Grand Central Publishing name and logo is a trademark of Hachette Book Group, Inc.

The Hachette Speakers Bureau provides a wide range of authors for speaking events. To find out more, go to www.HachetteSpeakersBureau.com or call (866) 376-6591.

The publisher is not responsible for websites (or their content) that are not owned by the publisher.

Library of Congress Cataloging-in-Publication Data

Heller, Marla.
   The DASH diet weight loss solution: 2 weeks to drop pounds, boost metabolism, and get healthy / Marla Heller. — 1st ed.
      p. cm.
   Includes bibliographical references and index.
   ISBN 978-1-4555-1279-9 (hardcover) — ISBN 978-1-4555-1278-2 (trade pbk.) — ISBN 978-1-4555-1277-5 (ebook)   1. Weight loss—Popular works.   2. Metabolism.   3. Nutrition.   4. Reducing diets—Recipes.   I. Title.
   RM222.2.H3618 2012
   613.2'5—dc23

                                                                2012027212

To my husband, Richard,
who always supports me,
and to my mom,
who taught me how to cook and make healthy, balanced meals.

CONTENTS

THE

DASH
DIET
Weight Loss
Solution

CHAPTER 1

Conquering Weight Loss—
The DASH Diet Weight Loss Solution

It's about time! The DASH diet has already been named the "Best Overall Diet" and the "Healthiest Diet" by *U.S. News & World Report*. Now *The DASH Diet Weight Loss Solution* turns it into America's best weight loss diet, as well. This plan is specifically designed to supercharge weight loss, giving you the boost you need to achieve your goals quickly, easily, and with results that will last. The health benefits of the DASH (Dietary Approaches to Stop Hypertension) diet are well known. It lowers blood pressure in 14 days. It lowers cholesterol and improves brain function. People who follow the DASH diet have lower rates of heart attack, stroke, heart failure, and some types of cancer, including BRCA negative breast cancer. Additionally, people who follow the DASH eating plan are less likely to develop diabetes or kidney stones.

The DASH diet has been one of the best-kept secrets

for healthy eating. And now, previously overlooked research provides the foundation for enhanced weight loss results. Based on scientific evidence, and the real world success I've personally seen with hundreds of clients, the program in *The DASH Diet Weight Loss Solution* attacks weight loss with the same efficiency and effectiveness that it attacks our nation's leading health problems. With this book, you can deploy DASH to help you reach and maintain a healthy weight.

You are already reading this book, so we know you are interested in reaching and maintaining a healthier weight. And you have chosen a diet plan that will actually make you healthier as you move toward your goal. Many quick weight loss plans are very difficult to follow in a normal, active life. Or the plans are great for initiating weight loss, but they aren't sustainable and wouldn't be healthy if you did sustain them for any period of time. *The DASH Diet Weight Loss Solution* is a plan that you and your family can follow for the long run. In fact, it is based on the 2010 Dietary Guidelines for Americans. It is a two-phase plan guaranteed to boost weight loss. Phase One is a two-week transition to reset your metabolism. This protein-rich eating plan will keep you satisfied longer and will help jump-start your weight loss, resulting in fast, visible results. Phase Two includes whole grains and fruits, as well as lots of nonstarchy vegetables and lean proteins, and will help you continue to lose weight. In addition to looking and feeling better, you will also improve your cholesterol, blood sugar levels, and blood pressure. The results have been proven and the research backs it up. You will also find detailed meal plans, pantry stocking advice, grocery shopping tips—and dozens of delicious recipes to incorporate into your diet.

What has the research shown?

Over 67% of Americans are overweight or obese. And excess weight is not just a cosmetic problem. The yearly direct health care costs for obesity hit $147 billion in 2008, accounting for almost 10% of all health care costs in the United States. On average, someone who is obese spends $1,500 per year extra for medical care than someone of healthy weight.

What are some of the health problems that are more common in people who carry too much weight? Health issues can include hypertension (high blood pressure); type 2 diabetes; joint problems; sleep apnea; coronary heart disease; elevated cholesterol and triglycerides; certain types of cancer; stroke; gall bladder; and liver diseases.

And extra weight by itself is limiting. Imagine picking up a 40-pound bag of dog food and carrying it around all day. Then visualize how good it will feel to set down the extra 40 pounds you have been hefting. The same thing will be true in real life when you drop your excess weight. All of your routine tasks will feel easier—and you will become more active.

Now you can take advantage of this supercharged version of the DASH diet to boost weight loss, especially the muffin top fat that is associated with increased risk for heart disease and diabetes. In the old days, we talked about apple body shapes being more unhealthful than the pear body shapes. Belly fat, beer bellies, visceral fat, android fat, and muffin top are just different words for people who carry much of their excess weight around the middle. This type of fat is associated with higher risks for diabetes, heart disease, high blood pressure, and some kinds of cancer.

Over the past two decades, much has been learned about

why this belly fat is different from other fat, and what kind of eating patterns are associated with it. The main culprits? Taking in more carbs than we can burn off, and having less metabolically active muscle. In this book we will target both of these problems, getting you unhooked from a carb-heavy diet, and helping you to increase your metabolism by preserving and strengthening muscles. No, we aren't massively bulking up (relax, ladies), but you will become leaner and more toned. You can reduce bad cholesterol and triglycerides while boosting good cholesterol. And perhaps most important for many people, the lower-starch version of the DASH diet can reduce the risk of developing diabetes or improve your ability to control your diabetes and slow the progression of the disease. All of this comes with reduced inflammation and oxidative stress.

Back in the 1990s, the prevailing healthy eating advice recommended high intake of carbs—maybe that was the pasta decade. It also recommended very low fat intake, and held that most people were consuming too much protein. What happened as a result of this advice? The "diabesity epidemic" (a coined term to reflect the interaction of diabetes and obesity) took hold and led to massive increases in poor health and health care costs.

To be more specific, in 1988, 26% of the population was obese, and by 2008, 40% were obese. The yearly costs of the related diseases are about $150 billion for obesity, $157 billion for diabetes, and $445 billion for heart disease. This is an overwhelming burden for our health care system. It is time for us to turn these statistics around and make ourselves healthier.

In this book we will help you take advantage of newer research regarding the benefits of reduced intake of refined grains and added sugars, the need for higher than previously recommended levels of protein, and strategies for preparing meals and snacks that are satisfying and actually help to curb hunger. And fortunately, these new concepts actually conform to the strategies from the forgotten lower-carb DASH study.

Why wasn't this newer information immediately pursued? It was very difficult for the traditional medical establishment to accept that their high-grain, low-fat, limited-protein diet recommendations were wrong, and were, in fact, doing great harm to the collective health of our country.

The combined benefits of the newer concepts for healthy eating, presented here, will help you find the easy way to lose weight, especially that muffin top. Even better, you will do this while learning an easy-to-sustain healthy way to eat.

Most fad diets promise quick weight loss. The DASH Diet Weight Loss Solution is great for speeding up weight loss. But we also show you how to become healthier in the process. And it is a plan you can all follow for a lifetime! In the next chapter, you will learn more about why the plan works.

Before moving forward, take a moment to assess your health goals. Where are you now and where do you want to be? Having a goal will help you to succeed—and you will be amazed by how quickly and easily you will meet your targets once you are living the DASH lifestyle.

Making My Personal DASH Diet Plan

What Are My Health Goals?

Healthier weight? _____
  Current _____ Target _____

Drop inches around my waist? _____
  Current _____ Target _____

Lower my blood pressure? _____
  Current _____ Target _____

Lower my cholesterol? _____
  Current _____ Target _____

Lower my triglycerides? _____
  Current _____ Target _____

Additional goals: _____

_____

CHAPTER 2

The DASH Diet Weight Loss Breakthrough

At the time that the DASH diet was first developed, in the mid-1990s, the prevailing nutrition wisdom was to encourage lots of grains and low-fat eating. But everyone got fatter and less healthy.

Next came the proliferation of low-carb diets. Because it was initially pooh-poohed by the medical establishment, imagine the surprise when research showed no adverse health effects from increased fat intake. With conventional dietary wisdom turned on its head, the DASH researchers designed a new study to evaluate the effects of lower-carb versions of the DASH eating program. In other words, they wanted to do their own side-by-side comparison to see if a DASH diet with some of the starches replaced with either higher levels of protein or more heart-healthy fats would provide the same health benefits as the original (higher-carb) DASH diet. And imagine their surprise when the blood pressure improvements were even better with the low-starch versions of DASH.

This is the first book to use the long-overlooked NIH-sponsored research and present the lower-starch version of the DASH diet. In combination with other research studies that have helped us learn about the weight loss and health benefits of lower-carb eating plans, you will now have the optimized plan in *The DASH Diet Weight Loss Solution*.

As a dietitian in private practice and at a naval hospital outpatient nutrition clinic, I have successfully implemented this new and improved DASH diet plan with hundreds of people. Many of these were military members who needed to lose weight to maintain fitness levels required by their branch of service. These sailors, soldiers, marines, and airmen needed to stay fit and healthy, and that would not have been possible with an unhealthy quick-fix plan. Yes, the new DASH diet plan sped up weight loss. But we met the weight goal while maintaining the muscle mass required for fitness. The result: improved metabolism, lower body fat, enhanced strength and cardiovascular fitness, and improved health.

The new DASH plan, specifically designed to speed weight loss, also proved effective for the families of military and for military retirees who had diabetes or prediabetes. Lowering blood glucose levels, reducing blood pressure, improving cholesterol and triglycerides, while reaching a healthier weight, became easy for these patients. The lower-carb DASH diet kept hunger under control with filling, low-calorie fruits and veggies, while providing long-lasting satiety with lean protein-rich foods and heart-healthy fats. With an abundance of great food, the lower-carb DASH diet did not feel like a diet at all.

Never before presented to the general public, The DASH Diet Weight Loss Solution is the perfect antidote to America's obesity epidemic. Still rich in the key DASH foods—fruits; vegetables; low-fat and nonfat dairy; lean meats, fish, and poultry; nuts, beans, and seeds; moderate amounts of whole grains; and heart-healthy fats—this DASH program improves the health benefits and provides quicker, more dramatic, sustainable weight loss than the original DASH eating plan, presented in my first book, *The DASH Diet Action Plan*.

Before going into the full-blown version of this new DASH diet, many people will benefit from going through a "reset" phase, to wipe out their cravings and jump-start their weight loss. So in Chapter 3, we have a surefire way to wake up your fat-burning metabolism and develop a cleaner way of eating that eliminates cravings.

How do you reconcile low-carb and the DASH diet? First, you don't need all the refined starchy foods that most of us overconsume. They are certainly not part of making the DASH diet a healthy plan.

And getting more of the protein-rich foods is important as we get older. Back in the late 1980s and early 1990s, the RDAs for protein were set very low. The target level was that which was needed to prevent muscle wasting during starvation. But it was not high enough to prevent muscle loss on aging. And nutrition professionals, at that time, were taught to make weight loss plans in which calories from all the food groups were lowered proportionally. Today we know that when you help people reduce their calories, you want to keep the protein level high enough to preserve muscle mass. It is primarily the carb calories that you want to reduce.

Certainly, whole grains are healthful. The fiber, lignans, vitamins, and minerals are beneficial. But we do have to be careful not to consume more than we can burn off. And often grains come in foods packed with sugars. From Barbara Rolls's research studies that resulted in the Volumetrics program, we know that foods that contain water are more filling than drier foods. Most of the grain foods, such as breads, pastries, cookies, dry cereals, and even popcorn, are relatively low in moisture. Since they are not filling, we are more likely to overeat these types of foods. A diet that "forgets" these refined grain foods actually makes it easier to curb calories without having to think about it too much.

Another reason why starchy foods tend to provoke hunger is that they break down rather quickly to sugar. More accurately, they break down to glucose. Glucose is the blood sugar that we monitor in diabetics. When there is a surge of glucose into the blood, it triggers the body to pump out insulin to regulate blood sugar. When we are younger and relatively fit, we respond well to the insulin, blood sugar does not go too high, and the glucose moves into our muscle tissue to provide energy for physical activity. However, as we get older, and if we are less fit, the muscles do not respond as well to insulin. The bad news is that our mid-body fat does respond well to insulin, so the sugar gets stored in our belly fat and is then converted into more fat. And it is possible for the insulin to overshoot its target, causing our blood sugar to drop, triggering even more hunger. These up-and-down spikes of blood sugar can lead to more cravings and feeling out of control with your hunger. Meals that are just based on starches and/or sugars will leave us feeling hungry again relatively quickly.

On the other hand, fruits and vegetables also contain carbohydrates. They are rich in fiber, contain naturally occurring sugars, and pack in lots of water, so that they are relatively low in calories for their size. Fruits and vegetables are bulky and filling, which makes these foods wonderful choices for filling your plate. And of course, they are rich in all kinds of vitamins, minerals, antioxidants, and other healthful plant nutrients. Some vegetables contain more starch and are more caloric than others, so we probably want to watch the portion sizes more carefully with these foods, such as potatoes, winter squash, and peas. But with all the rest, an abundance makes it much easier to stay on track.

Protein-rich foods are also more satisfying than foods made from refined grains. Protein takes longer to digest, and it doesn't cause the blood sugar spike of the starchy foods. You are much more likely to feel full longer if you add some protein-rich foods to your meals and snacks. With *The DASH Diet Weight Loss Solution*, you will learn to mix it up. For example, if you have a snack with fruit and some light cheese or a handful of nuts, you will feel full longer. Include a hard-boiled egg at breakfast. If you are having some pasta, be sure to add a meat sauce or beans to make the meal more satisfying. We need more protein as we get older. Our goal as we age is to keep as much muscle as possible.

Heart-healthy fats are also an important part of the mix in providing satiety. Fats slow down digestion so that energy from your food enters your bloodstream more slowly. Yes, fats have more calories than carbs or protein. However, in moderate quantities they are very beneficial for keeping hunger under control. Often when recipes reduce the amount of fat in the food, they don't reduce the calories. How can this happen? One of the things that fats do in recipes is to help hold in air introduced during mixing. So without the fat, the food is denser, and a serving might have the same calories with or without the fat. Remember the low-fat cookies popular in the early 1990s? They had exactly the same amount of calories as the full-fat cookies they replaced. Life isn't fair. But that does provide another example of where the high-carb, low-fat diets went awry.

What about the health issues around fats, carbs, and protein?

In the 1980s and 1990s, it was generally believed that low-fat, low-protein, high-carb diets were best for heart health. The experts told us that diets higher in fat would cause our cholesterol and triglycerides to soar. Higher protein would cause our kidneys to fail. However, in actuality, the high-carb diets can cause triglycerides to spike, especially if someone is insulin resistant. Elevated triglycerides can be an early sign of impending type 2 diabetes. And high-carb diets tend to stoke the production of bad cholesterol, while depressing the level of good cholesterol.

Research has shown that people who consume heart-healthy fats, especially olive oil, nuts, and seafood rich in DHA and EPA, have lower rates of cardiovascular mortality. Add in their anti-inflammatory properties and these heart-healthy fats are definitely on our must-have list.

It was once thought that high-protein diets would be bad for everyone since excess protein would create extra work for the kidneys. However, we are not recommending excessively high levels of protein. And of course, traditional diets with high levels of salt, sugar, and starch do create extra work for the kidneys, and elevated blood sugar can harm the small blood vessels of the kidneys. Fortunately, the balanced approach of the DASH Diet Weight Loss Solution is consistent with heart health and is less likely to aggravate the kidneys than the traditional American diet. Of course, people with existing kidney disease who have been told to follow certain dietary restrictions by their physician or dietitian should check with their health care professional before adopting any new eating plan.

Another theorized health concern was that high-protein diets might impact bone health. Newer research shows that moderate intake of protein is associated with improved bone health and reduced risk for bone thinning as compared with a lower-protein diet.

Weighty Issues

With this book, you will learn that the most important things that you can do to lose weight are to get on track with healthy eating and become more physically active. Not only will you be healthier, but you will feel better and look better, too.

What Is a Healthy Weight?

There are many definitions of what makes a healthy weight, but the most obvious one is the weight at which you have no health problems. And unfortunately, even individuals whose weight fits the definition of "healthy" can still have habits—such as eating too many processed foods and being inactive—that are causing them to be at increased risk for certain diseases. This is called "metabolic obesity" or "normal weight obesity."

Currently, BMI (Body Mass Index) is the most common measure used to define healthy weight. If BMI is between 19 and 24, it is considered to be healthy. Between 25 and 29 is considered overweight. BMI over 30 is considered to be obese, and in excess of 40 is extreme obesity. These categories aren't just arbitrary distinctions. Health risks go up in each category. For example, women in the overweight category are about 70% more likely to have high blood pressure, compared with normal weight women, and twice as likely if they are obese. The concerns are much more dramatic with diabetes, with women who have a BMI over 35 being 30 times more likely to develop the disease, and even women who are just in the overweight category having about 18 times higher risk for diabetes.

Now, BMI cannot tell you how fit you are, and it is certainly possible for someone to have a BMI in the obese category, but not actually be "overfat." Football players, for example, are normally very muscular and will have weights that appear to be too high by BMI standards. But they are likely to be very fit. A measure of fitness could be percent body fat. This can be evaluated through underwater weighing, DEXA x-ray evaluation, bioelectrical impedance (BIA) done by professional equipment with electrodes, or even home scales that perform BIA to give a percent body fat reading.

Waist size is a very simple measure of whether your weight is healthy. If your waist is over 35 inches (88 cm) for women or over 40 inches (102 cm) for men, there are health concerns that you will want to have evaluated. You may have elevated blood pressure, blood sugar, and/or triglycerides. Even if your BMI is in the healthy zone, with too much belly fat you need to change your eating habits and start to exercise more. Fortunately, the DASH Diet Weight Loss Solution attacks this mid-body fat. At one time, no one believed in being able to "spot reduce." However, since excess belly fat is mostly due to overconsumption of starches and sugars, following this program will help you lose your muffin top.

Your Healthy Weight Goal

Setting targets, and especially short-term targets, can be very motivating and help keep you on track. Your weight target should fall somewhere in the healthy to overweight categories. If you have a lot to lose, setting a more modest goal, say, 5% to 10% of your current weight, would help you feel successful as you meet and exceed your targets, and make you healthier. In the Diabetes Prevention Study, losing as little as 7% of body weight significantly lowered the risk of diabetes.

BMI (Body Mass Index)

Height (inches)	18	19	20	21	22	23	24	25	26	27	28	29	30	31	32	33	34	35	36	37	38	39	40
58	86	91	96	100	105	110	115	120	124	129	134	139	144	148	153	158	163	167	172	177	182	187	191
59	89	94	99	104	109	114	119	124	129	134	139	144	149	153	158	163	168	173	178	183	188	193	198
60	92	97	102	108	113	118	123	128	133	138	143	148	154	159	164	169	174	179	184	189	195	200	205
61	95	101	106	111	116	122	127	132	138	143	148	153	159	164	169	175	180	185	191	196	201	206	212
62	98	104	109	115	120	126	131	137	142	148	153	158	164	169	175	180	186	191	197	202	208	213	219
63	102	107	113	119	124	130	135	141	147	152	158	163	169	175	180	186	192	198	203	209	215	220	226
64	105	111	117	122	128	134	140	146	151	157	163	169	175	181	186	192	198	204	210	216	221	227	233
65	108	114	120	126	132	138	144	150	156	162	168	174	180	186	192	198	204	210	216	222	228	234	240
66	112	118	124	130	136	142	149	155	161	167	173	180	186	192	198	204	211	217	223	229	235	242	248
67	115	121	128	134	140	147	153	160	166	172	179	185	192	198	204	211	217	223	230	236	243	249	255
68	118	125	132	138	145	151	158	164	171	178	184	191	197	204	210	217	224	230	237	243	250	256	263
69	122	129	135	142	149	156	163	169	176	183	190	196	203	210	217	223	230	237	244	251	257	264	271
70	125	132	139	146	153	160	167	174	181	188	195	202	209	216	223	230	237	244	251	258	265	272	279
71	129	136	143	151	158	165	172	179	186	194	201	208	215	222	229	237	244	251	258	265	272	280	287
72	133	140	147	155	162	170	177	184	192	199	206	214	221	229	236	243	251	258	265	273	280	288	295
73	136	144	152	159	167	174	182	189	197	205	212	220	227	235	243	250	258	265	273	280	288	296	303
74	140	148	156	164	171	179	187	195	203	210	218	226	234	241	249	257	265	273	280	288	296	304	312
75	144	152	160	168	176	184	192	200	208	216	224	232	240	248	256	264	272	280	288	296	304	312	320
76	148	156	164	173	181	189	197	205	214	222	230	238	246	255	263	271	279	288	296	304	312	320	329
77	152	160	169	177	186	194	202	211	219	228	236	245	253	261	270	278	287	295	304	312	320	329	337
78	156	164	173	182	190	199	208	216	225	234	242	251	260	268	277	286	294	303	312	320	329	337	346
79	160	169	178	186	195	204	213	222	231	240	249	257	266	275	284	293	302	311	320	328	337	346	355
80	164	173	182	191	200	209	218	228	237	246	255	264	273	282	291	300	309	319	328	337	346	355	364
81	168	177	187	196	205	215	224	233	243	252	261	271	280	289	299	308	317	327	336	345	355	364	373
82	172	182	191	201	210	220	230	239	249	258	268	277	287	296	306	316	325	335	344	354	363	373	383

Code: BMI under 19: Underweight   BMI 19–24: Healthy weight   BMI 25–29 Overweight
BMI 30–39: Obesity   BMI 40 and above: Extreme obesity

What are your personal health risks?

- Waist size too large? ❏
- Blood pressure too high? ❏
- Cholesterol or triglycerides too high? ❏
- High-salt diet? ❏
- Eating too many sugary or starchy foods? ❏
- Eating too many fried foods? ❏
- Not eating enough vegetables? ❏ fruit? ❏ dairy? ❏

We are *not* going to calculate your target calories. That's right, you will not need to count calories. Instead you will focus on including food groups, and learn to watch portion sizes, especially for the high-calorie foods. This is so much simpler. After all, we eat food, not calories. Focusing on how to include a variety of food groups will teach you habits that you will use for a lifetime.

Further, you want to be sure that you are losing fat, not muscle. A balanced plan with plenty of protein, calcium, and magnesium will help preserve muscle. Adding exercise, especially strength training, will also help with maintaining lean body mass and help keep metabolism as high as possible.

The DASH Diet Weight Loss Solution

With this plan, you will stay full, crave less junk food, and feel like you are eating in a way that is cleaner and lighter. You will want to continue to have this feeling. This makes it much easier to stay on track with your plan.

During the first phase, you will relearn how to make meals. Your focus will be on choosing protein-rich foods that add satiety. You will learn to pair the protein foods with vegetables that provide bulk and happen to be very healthy and very low-calorie. This phase will reset your taste preferences, and turn you on to lighter, healthier eating. It is a two-week transition to reset your entire approach to eating. And it will boost weight loss. The faster, initial weight loss is very motivating, because of the visible changes. You will quickly notice that your clothes fit looser, especially around the waist.

The only key DASH diet component that is missing during phase one is fruit. The good news is that it is missing only during the first phase. We are giving your digestive hormones, liver, and pancreas a break from your typical diet. It is especially important to allow your blood sugar to be calm and stable. By not including starchy and sugary foods, you will ensure that you won't have blood sugar spikes. You will avoid the highs and lows that are typical of most eating patterns. This immediately calms your hunger.

Other side benefits that have been reported during the initial phase include reduction or elimination of gastric reflux, reduced "brain fog," and reduced symptoms of allergies. Because there are no grains, of course, this part of the plan is gluten-free. It does contain dairy since that is a key part of the DASH diet, but you can also choose dairy substitutes if that is a problem for you.

After this initial reset phase, you are ready for Phase Two, which is a lower-carb plan. You will have already learned to make your meals more satisfying with proteins, nonstarchy vegetables, and heart-healthy fats. In Phase Two, you get to add whole grains and fruits. You will continue to lose weight, although slightly more slowly after the initial reset phase. This becomes a plan that you can enjoy for the rest of your life.

PART I

Developing Your Own DASH Diet Solution

Phase One: 2 Weeks to Reset Your Metabolism, Turbocharge Weight Loss, and Shrink Your Waistline

The DASH Diet Weight Loss Solution does not require you to count calories. You will, however, focus on getting a balance of food groups. We will mainly have a positive focus on foods you want to include rather than spending too much time on what you should avoid.

During Phase One, you will follow a more restrictive diet than in Phase Two, but this will help you develop the eating habits that will make you very successful with DASH. These habits will help you reach your weight loss goal and maintain that healthy weight. What are these key habits? First, you will learn to consume lots of vegetables and to rely on them for bulk in your diet. You will also learn to include protein-rich foods that increase satiety, help reduce in-between-meal hunger, and keep your blood sugar more stable. Without starchy and sugary foods, your metabolism will operate more efficiently, since you will have a reduced demand for insulin. You will notice that you are eating much lighter and cleaner, which will feel good. Within the first few days, you will also notice that your waist is shrinking because you are losing belly fat. People who have frequent complaints of heartburn may notice that they are not experiencing problems on this plan.

If you have diabetes and are on medication for it, please consult with your physician and/or dietitian about adopting this plan. It can significantly reduce your need for medication. But do not alter your medication intake without consulting first with your health care professional. This is also true for your blood pressure. If you find that your blood pressure is low, please contact your doctor before changing your blood pressure medication dosage.

During the first phase, you will improve your metabolism, and your need for insulin will drop significantly. While insulin promotes muscle development in children, in adults it promotes fat storage. With almost no starch or sugar during this phase, you will stop feeding the belly fat. Along with noticeable weight loss will come a reduction in waist size. Insulin can also trigger hunger. With less insulin circulating, and a more stable blood sugar, your hunger will finally get under control.

Many people who struggle with weight and health issues have what is known as metabolic syndrome (also called dysmetabolic syndrome, or Syndrome X). Women with PCOS (polycystic ovary syndrome) may have metabolic syndrome. It is related to a combination of symptoms, including elevated triglycerides, blood pressure, blood sugar, and waist circumference, and/or low HDL. Current estimates suggest that 25% of

Americans have this syndrome. Fortunately, the DASH Diet Weight Loss Solution addresses all of these symptoms. In addition to your waist size shrinking, your blood pressure should become more normal, along with your triglycerides, HDL, and blood sugar.

As I mentioned earlier, instead of counting calories, you focus on including the key food groups. How does that work? During the first phase, you will learn to fill your plate with low-calorie vegetables and sufficient protein to make the meal satisfying. This instantly reduces your normal mealtime demand for insulin, and keeps your blood sugar on a more even keel.

Phase One: The Intuitive 14-Day Plan

Our ultrasimple introduction will provide you with an overview of how Phase One works. Sample meal plans will be found in Chapter 4. Many people are trying to avoid foods that are highly processed or that contain artificial sweeteners, while others prefer quick and easy. Substitutions are provided to accommodate both preferences here. This plan will work for everyone.

Include Moderate-Sized Servings of These Foods

Foods That Are Protein-Rich and Low in Saturated Fat

- Lean meats, fish, and poultry
- Beans, lentils, soy foods
- Low-fat or nonfat cheeses
- Egg substitutes and some whole eggs if desired
- Unsweetened or artificially sweetened yogurt (one per day)

Heart-Healthy Fats

- Avocados
- Vegetable oils, especially olive oil, canola oil, and nut oils. (Coconut oil and palm oil are excluded, since they are high in saturated fat.)
- Salad dressings, especially those based on the above oils

Foods That Are Protein-Rich and Contain Healthy Fat

- Nuts (preferably nonroasted and unsalted) and seeds
- Fatty fish

Enjoy as Much of These Foods as You Want

- Infused water, such as with fruit slices or herbs. However, in Phase 1 don't eat the fruit slices.
- Nonstarchy vegetables. (Exclusions include potatoes, winter squash, corn, etc.)
- Sugar-free gelatin. (optional)

Avoid These Foods

- Starchy foods (other than beans). This means no bread, pasta, potatoes, rice, etc. No foods fried in batter.
- Sugary foods, including fruit
- Alcohol
- Milk
- Caffeinated beverages other than with meals or snacks

Seven Steps to Success

1. *Do not skip any meals or snacks.* This will keep your blood sugar steady, and help you avoid hunger. People who think that they will speed up the weight loss by skipping meals or snacks have reported feeling shaky

or light-headed. Your goal is to learn how your hunger is easily controlled when your blood sugar is more modulated.

2. *Limit exercise to no more than 30 minutes of light or moderate activity per day during the initial phase; you do not want to drive your blood sugar too low.* While exercise is not essential during Phase One, we know that moderate activity such as walking helps with burning belly fat, without burning off muscle.

3. *Go to sleep earlier.* You will feel less energetic during the "jump start," and will find yourself wanting to go to sleep earlier than normal. This is okay; don't worry about it. Your energy level will go back to normal at the end of the first two weeks.

4. *Don't be overly restrictive with salt, and get plenty of fluids, at least eight glasses per day.* (Yes, even caffeinated beverages count, as does the gelatin.) This will help boost energy. The initial 14-day program can be dehydrating. Without starchy and sugary foods in your diet, your body will flush out excess fluid. Allowing yourself to have a moderate amount of salty foods will help prevent too much fluid loss.

5. *Tell yourself that you just need to stick with the program "today."* You can stick with the plan for just one meal, then another, and then another to get through one day. Build a series of these days to complete the two weeks. The one-meal-, one-day-at-a-time philosophy does work.

6. *Try to relax.* You may get cranky in the middle of the jump-start period. It is not unheard of for someone to have a mini-"meltdown" in the middle of this phase. Walk away and try to relax. Your body is going through a lot of changes, all for the better. Keep going; it will get easier tomorrow.

7. *Focus on your weight loss results.* Your success will keep you focused and make it easier to stay on track. It is absolutely okay to weigh yourself daily, especially during this phase; it will build an aura of success. For women, you may find that your weight loss gets a little stalled at the end of the second week. Don't worry about this; it will pick up again when you start the next phase.

Phase One Eating

In Chapter 4, you will find detailed menus for the next 14 days. Below, though, are general guidelines and suggestions when preparing meals during Phase One.

Breakfasts
- Egg whites or egg substitutes. May top with some light cheese. (May use whole eggs 1–2 days a week.)
- 1–2 slices lean meats, which may include Canadian bacon or ham, or soy alternatives
- Tomato juice or V8 juice if desired
- Egg alternatives: the lunchtime roll-ups, or yogurt without added sugar

Midmorning Snacks
At least two of the following:
- Low-fat cheese, such as cheeses made from 2% milk, light string cheese, or light cottage cheese (4-ounce size)
- Veggies, including celery, radishes, carrots, cucumbers, sliced peppers, grape or cherry tomatoes

- Nuts, ¼ cup or less. If having nuts and cheese, limit nuts to 1 tablespoon.

Lunches

Choose one of the protein-rich main courses, and all of the other side dishes.

- Salad loaded with a variety of veggies and protein foods. No croutons. Although light cheese is preferred, you can occasionally have regular cheese.
- Stuffed tomato with egg salad, egg white salad, chicken salad, and/or tuna salad
- Roll-ups made with ham, turkey, or lean roast beef and low-fat cheese and/or lettuce as the wrap
- Veggies and/or side salad with dressing
- Sugar-free Jell-O

Midafternoon Snacks (and Before-Dinner Snack, If Needed)

Same as the morning snacks. Additional choices include:

- Pepper strips dipped in guacamole or salad dressing
- Peanuts in the shell. A serving is 10, which would be 20 individual peanuts.

Dinners

Include all of the following:

- Lean meat, fish, poultry, or meat substitute
- Nonstarchy veggies
- Salad with dressing
- Infused water, or optionally, flavored gelatin without added sugar

Dining Out Suggestions

Breakfasts

- Eggs or omelets
- Some bacon is okay.
- Tomato or V8 juice (6 ounces or less)

Hint: Instead of toast and/or potatoes, ask if you can have sliced tomatoes.

Lunches

- Salads topped with lean protein-rich food
- Burger or chicken without the bun, with side vegetables and/or salad or coleslaw

Hint: Eating burgers without the bun will become a habit. Remember, there is no rule against having vegetables (other than French fries) with a burger. Ask what kinds of side veggies are available. The salads work for fast-food options, or get a side salad and cut up the burger or chicken for your salad—without the bun.

Dinners

- Lean meat, fish, or poultry
- Side vegetables
- Side salad with dressing

Hint: Leave before dessert.

Hit the Grocery Store to Stock Up On…

- Individually packaged light cheeses such as: Cheeses made from 2% milk, light string cheese, and light cottage cheese (4-ounce size)

- Eggs or egg substitute
- Sugar-free Jell-O packages (optional)
- Sliced light cheese and lean deli meats
- Nuts, preferably not roasted in oil. Examples are ball-park peanuts, dry-roasted or raw almonds, cashews, or walnuts. Choose nuts that are not addictive for you. Nuts in the shell slow you down, which will help you avoid overdoing it.
- Guacamole
- Canned tuna, salmon, or other fatty fish
- Extra-lean ground sirloin
- Beef cuts such as round, chuck, or with "loin" in the name
- Skinless chicken breasts
- Lean pork chops, pork loin, or tenderloin
- Turkey breasts
- Fish and other seafood (not breaded or fried)
- Fresh vegetables such as lettuce, fresh peppers, baby carrots, radishes, tomatoes, zucchini, summer squash, jicama, etc.
- Frozen vegetables (without sauce) such as broccoli, mixed vegetables, green beans, peas, cauliflower, spinach, Brussels sprouts, etc.
- For vegetarians, soy foods including tofu, dry beans, or lentils.

Note: Please choose the foods you like from the above list. This plan would be much too hard if you were trying to eat foods that you hate.

Fast and Easy Tips

Check out the salad bar for sliced peppers, cucumbers, radishes, celery, etc., and for salads.

Hit the deli counter for coleslaw; egg, tuna, and chicken salads; and poached salmon.

Pick up a rotisserie chicken or roasted turkey breast from the ready-to-eat section.

Stock up on ready-made Jell-O cups (artificially sweetened).

Plan, Plan, Plan

- Take your lunches and snacks to work. Either stock your fridge at the office, or bring an insulated bag with all the right foods.
- Make sure you keep all the key DASH foods on hand.
- Do not skip any meals or snacks.
- Plan what you will eat for each meal and snack, each day.
- Cook foods ahead for quick meals.
  - On weekends, grill several chicken breasts, which can be used for other meals, as salad toppings, or for chicken salad.
  - Make lots of hard-boiled eggs. Peel, and pop into zipper bags to store in the fridge. Use for quick breakfasts, salad toppings, egg salad, or tuna salad.
  - Grill several burgers on the weekend, to use for quick meals.
  - Make chili, spaghetti, or sloppy joes to use for several meals.
- Plan what you will eat before you go into a restaurant.

Remember your goal. Then plan to succeed.

Overview of Phase One Diet Patterns

The following table will help you understand the daily food group patterns for the DASH Diet Weight Loss Solution, Phase One.

Phase One Food Group Servings per Day			
	Smaller appetite	*Moderate appetite*	*Larger appetite*
Nonstarchy vegetables	Unlimited, minimum of 5		
Dairy	2	2–3	2–4
Nuts, beans, seeds	1	1–2	1–2
Lean meat, fish, poultry, eggs	5–6 ounces	6–8 ounces	8–11 ounces
Fats	1–2	2–3	2–4

What will you have accomplished?

During Phase One, you will have learned to fill your plate with lots of colorful vegetables, and to complement them with lean meats, fish, and poultry or other protein-rich foods, and you will have added low-fat dairy to your regimen. You will have also learned that your hunger is easy to manage when your blood sugar doesn't have highs and lows. And you will have calmed your body's response to your previous intake of excess calories, especially the sugars and starches. Your body won't be overproducing triglycerides and LDL cholesterol, or the fat storage hormone, insulin. As a result, you will lose weight and feel great! What a great start to a weight loss plan that will improve your health, and be easy to follow. It is a new way of eating, one that will become your way of eating for a lifetime.

My Actions to Get Started with the DASH Diet Weight Loss Solution

I will go to the grocery store to buy the right foods.

Key new foods for me will be: _____

Key favorites for me will be: _____

Challenges that might interfere for me: _____
_____

How I will deal with these challenges: _____
_____

CHAPTER 4

14 Days of Metabolism-Boosting Menus

Our ultrasimple diet instructions in Chapter 3 provide virtually everything you need to know to follow Phase One. Even better, you will enjoy seeing a variety of ways to put together the meals and snacks. It can be much easier to get on track with a new eating plan if you can visualize how everything fits together. In this chapter you will be provided with a sample 14-day menu plan. These meals are just suggestions. You can substitute similar types of foods for any of the meals or snacks, or you can repeat any days that are particularly easy to follow or suit your taste preferences. You may also want to repeat dinners if you are cooking for one or two. It is absolutely fine to choose meals or snacks from any of the days and match up with meals from other days.

Remember, you do not want to skip any meals or snacks, and you want to have a balance of the bulky, filling foods along with the protein-rich foods. If you start to feel a little light-headed or dizzy, have another snack (or make sure you had the snack in the first place).

You are probably wondering about portion sizes. Filling your plate with lots of vegetables helps to provide satisfying meals. It is hard to go overboard on the nonstarchy vegetables. When you think about portion size for meats, fish, and poultry, at dinner try to choose a portion that is about the size of your palm. Larger men need more protein than smaller women, and will have larger palms. It is relatively proportional to your appropriate amount of protein. As you go through the initial phase, you will find that your appetite decreases. Stop eating when you have had enough and are comfortably satisfied. However, if you find that you are getting hungry shortly after meals, then your serving sizes are too small, especially the protein part. There is also a certain amount of boredom that will set in toward the end of the first 14 days. That is normal, and actually helps to keep your appetite under control.

Where possible, we have tried to suggest foods that require minimal preparation time by you. For example, for your side salads, you can use bagged mixes, such as a romaine mix, a spring mix, an iceberg mix, grated carrots, coleslaw blend, or broccoli slaw. Or you could combine some of these mixes and top romaine with one of the slaws. Hitting a salad bar at the grocery store would be another quick, low-prep way to add variety to your salads, and a great place to pick up hard-boiled eggs.

Speaking of eggs, there are a lot of eggs and egg substitutes in the plan. When choosing eggs, the ones that are high in omega-3s are good, since they are also reduced in cholesterol. And even the American Heart Association says that one regular, large egg per day fits into a heart-healthy diet.

We also have used some brand names in the menu plans, as they are easily recognizable. Do not feel that this is an endorsement of any of the brands. You may use any substitutes that you like, as long as they have similar nutritional properties.

Other than juices, we have not specified beverages in this part of the plan. Your choices include water, black coffee, unsweetened or artificially sweetened tea, and diet sodas. Do not have any alcoholic beverages. They may contain sugars, they definitely contain calories, and they do a very good job of reducing willpower and leading you down the path to diet ruination. So no alcohol in this phase!

Meal items that are marked with an asterisk (*) have associated recipes in Chapter 16.

Day 1

Breakfast

- Hard-boiled egg. Hint: Make several hard-boiled eggs, and peel. Store in a zipper bag in the refrigerator. Then you will have them when you need them, for super-quick breakfasts. You can also find prepackaged, peeled hard-boiled eggs in some stores. I like the Eggland's Best version, since they are lower in cholesterol and I think they have better taste.
- 1 or 2 slices Canadian bacon
- 6 ounces tomato juice, low-sodium

Midmorning Snack

- 1 stick light cheese
- Baby carrots

Lunch

- Acapulco Tuna Salad*
- Cherry tomatoes
- Small side salad: dressed with Italian or oil and vinegar dressing
- Infused water with orange slices, or sugar-free gelatin

Midafternoon Snack

- 4 ounces lemon light yogurt, fat-free, without added sugar
- 18 cashews (1 ounce by weight, ¼ cup by volume, or small handful)

Before-Dinner Snack (Optional)

- Pepper strips. Hint: To make the strips quickly, cut off the tops and bottoms of some red, yellow, or orange bell peppers. Remove seeds and cut in half. Flatten each half and take a very sharp knife and cut along the surface, removing the membranes. Then cut into 1-inch strips. These are great to dip into guacamole, as a chip substitute.
- 2 ounces guacamole, which is about ¼ cup

Dinner

- Crispy Grilled Chicken*
- 1 cup (or more) mixed carrots, broccoli, and cauliflower blend: steamed or microwaved
- Salad: romaine blend with Italian dressing
- Infused water with lemon slices

Day 2

Breakfast

- Mini omelet. You can liven this up with some diced red bell pepper (left over from last night?) or sliced grape tomatoes. Spray microwave-safe dish or cup with cooking spray. Add 1–2 eggs or egg whites and vegetables. Microwave on high for 1 minute. Stir, and cook an additional 15 seconds.
- 4–6 ounces tomato juice, low-sodium

Midmorning Snack

- 0.8–1 ounce 2% cheese, such as Swiss
- 6 grape tomatoes

Lunch

- 2–3 Turkey-Swiss roll-ups. Cheese on the outside, as the wrap. Deli or home-roasted turkey slices for the meat. Add whatever condiments you like, such as mustard. You could also add lettuce as the outermost layer of the wrap.
- ½–1 cup coleslaw
- Raw snow peas or sugar snap pea pods (as much as you like)
- Infused water with cucumber slices, and/or sugar-free gelatin

Midafternoon Snack

- 1 stick light 2% cheese
- Baby carrots

Before-Dinner Snack (Optional)

- 10 peanuts in the shell (20 individual peanuts) Hint: Shelling nuts slows you down, so you are less likely to overeat them.

Dinner

- Roasted sliced turkey
- Sautéed carrots and onions. Sauté 1 medium onion, thinly sliced, in 1 tablespoon olive oil or canola oil. Add about 8 ounces sliced carrots, and continue to sauté until the carrots are soft. Add 1 thin pat of butter at the end. Hints: Top the turkey with the sautéed carrots for extra flavor. If you like very soft carrots, microwave first before sautéing.
- Side salad topped with Italian dressing
- Infused water with lemon slices, and/or unsweetened gelatin

Day 3

Breakfast

- Scrambled eggs
- 1–2 slices Canadian bacon
- 4–6 ounces diet cranberry juice

Midmorning Snack

- 4 ounces raspberry light yogurt, nonfat, without added sugar
- 23 almonds (1 ounce by weight, ¼ cup by volume)

Lunch

- Cold fried chicken breast (don't eat the skin or coating) Hint: The chicken doesn't have to be cold. This could be a fast-food lunch but only if you can choose whole chicken parts. (Definitely, do not choose chicken tenders, patties, crispy chicken, or nuggets—too much breading for the amount of meat.) Most fried chicken places have coleslaw as a side. When you get back to your office, you can have the carrots and gelatin, if desired.

- Coleslaw
- Baby carrots
- Water, and/or gelatin without added sugar (optional)

Midafternoon Snack

- 1–2 slices 2% cheese
- 6 grape tomatoes

Before-Dinner Snack (Optional)

- Pepper strips
- Guacamole

Dinner

- Super-Savory Sliders*
- 1 cup broccoli
- Side salad with balsamic dressing
- Water infused with lime slices, and/or flavored gelatin without added sugar

Day 4

Breakfast

- Turkey-Swiss roll-up. 2% Swiss cheese as the wrap for 1–2 ounces turkey.
- 4–6 ounces tomato juice, low-sodium

Midmorning Snack

- 2 tablespoons chunky peanut butter
- 8 baby carrots

Lunch

- Salad with grilled chicken
- 20 walnuts
- Water infused with a sprig of rosemary, and/or flavored gelatin without added sugar

Midafternoon Snack

- 1 light string cheese stick
- Celery sticks

Before-Dinner Snack (Optional)

- Pepper strips
- Hummus

Dinner

- ¼ rotisserie chicken (precooked, from grocery store) or Stand-up Chicken*
- 1 cup peas (microwave from frozen)
- Side salad (from grocery store salad bar) with Italian dressing
- Water infused with lemon slices, and/or flavored gelatin without added sugar

Hint: This is a great dinner when you don't have a lot of preparation time. And yet it is a complete, hot meal.

Day 5

Breakfast

- Quick mini-omelet. Spray microwave-safe cup or dish with cooking spray. Add 1 or 2 eggs. Microwave on high for 1 minute. Stir, and heat for an additional 15 seconds.
- Diet cranberry juice or water infused with orange slices (optional)

Midmorning Snack

- 1 ounce 2% or light cheese
- Baby carrots

Lunch

- 2–3 Provolone cheese and roast beef roll-ups. Use the cheese as the wrap for the deli-sliced roast beef, or add a piece of lettuce for the outside wrap. Use mayo or mustard as the condiment, if desired.
- Italian coleslaw. Use bagged coleslaw and add very thin strips of red pepper and some grated carrots. Dress with Italian or other oil and vinegar dressing.
- Sliced tomato
- Water infused with cucumber, and/or flavored sugar-free gelatin

Midafternoon Snack

- 4-ounce strawberry-banana light yogurt, nonfat, without added sugar
- 10 cashews

Before-Dinner Snack (Optional)

- 20 pistachios in the shell. Hint: The shells slow you down.

Dinner

- Garden Splendor, Sautéed Chicken with Tomatoes over Haricots Verts*
- Caprese salad. 1 ounce sliced fresh mozzarella ball, alternated with 1 sliced medium tomato, dressed with 1 tablespoon olive oil and 1 tablespoon balsamic vinegar, and topped with 1 basil leaf, cut into very thin strips (*chiffonade*).
- Water infused with basil strips, and/or flavored gelatin without added sugar

Day 6

Breakfast

- 1–2 hard-boiled eggs
- 1 slice Canadian bacon
- 4–6 ounces tomato juice, low-sodium

Midmorning Snack

- 1 ounce light cheese
- Grape tomatoes

Lunch

- Salmon salad: Mix flaked, canned salmon with mayonnaise, celery, and/or other crunchy vegetables per your taste preferences.
- Sliced tomato

- Side salad with Italian dressing
- Water infused with lime slices, and/or flavored gelatin without added sugar

Midafternoon Snack

- Key lime light yogurt, nonfat, without added sugar
- Baby carrots

Before-Dinner Snack (Optional)

- 10 peanuts in the shell (20 individual peanuts)

Dinner

- Stand-up Chicken*
- Creamy Cauliflower Mashed Potatoes*
- Spinach
- Large tossed salad: Include iceberg and romaine lettuces, tomatoes, red cabbage, grated carrots, and pepper strips. Toss with an oil and vinegar or Italian or balsamic dressing.
- Water infused with cucumber slices, and/or flavored gelatin without added sugar

Hint: The Stand-up Chicken will take about an hour and 10 minutes to cook. So after you pop it in the oven, go for a walk or do some kind of activity.

Day 7

Breakfast

- Hard-boiled egg(s)
- 10 cashews
- 4–6 ounces tomato juice, low-sodium

Midmorning Snack

- 1 light string cheese stick
- Baby carrots

Lunch

- Buffalo chicken salad. Hint: This is a meal you could have in a restaurant. You have choices. Order yours with the chicken grilled instead of fried. Or you can make it yourself with grilled chicken, topped with hot sauce, and placed on top of your salad.
- Water infused with lemon slices, and/or flavored gelatin without added sugar

Midafternoon Snack

- Pineapple upside down cake light yogurt, nonfat, without added sugar
- 10 almonds

Before-Dinner Snack (Optional)

- Celery sticks
- Guacamole

Dinner

- Hearty Extra Veggie Chili,* topped with light shredded cheese and onions, if desired
- Black cherry Jell-O cup, sugar-free

Day 8

Breakfast

- 4 ounces reduced-fat cottage cheese
- Diet cranberry juice or water infused with orange slices

Midmorning Snack

- Strawberry shortcake light yogurt, nonfat, without added sugar

Lunch

- Cheeseburger. Hint: If from a restaurant, pitch the bun and cut up the burger to have on a salad or order it without the bun. Use whatever condiments you choose.
- Broccoli (if at a sit-down restaurant)
- Side salad with dressing
- Water infused with lime slices, and/or flavored gelatin without added sugar

Midafternoon Snack

- 1 light string cheese stick
- 20 walnuts

Before-Dinner Snack (Optional)

- Cut-up raw veggies
- Light ranch dip

Dinner

- Pan-seared salmon, coated with salt-free Cajun seasoning mix
- Sautéed peppers and onions. Hint: You could use a frozen mix, or cut up your own. Sauté in olive oil.

- Side salad with Italian or oil and vinegar dressing
- Water infused with cucumber slices, and/or flavored gelatin without added sugar

Day 9

Breakfast

- Quick mini cheese omelet. Spray microwave-safe dish or cup with cooking spray. Mix 1–2 eggs with 1 ounce light shredded cheese. Microwave on high for 1 minute, stir, then heat for an additional 15 seconds.
- 4–6 ounces diet cranberry juice

Midmorning Snack

- 1–2 light string cheese sticks
- 8 baby carrots

Lunch

- Turkey and Swiss roll-ups (2–3)
- Coleslaw
- Cherry tomatoes
- Raspberry Jell-O cup, sugar-free
- Water infused with lemon slices, and/or flavored gelatin without added sugar

Midafternoon Snack

- Strawberry light yogurt, nonfat, without added sugar
- 10 cashews

Before-Dinner Snack (Optional)

- Pepper strips
- ¼ cup guacamole

Dinner

- Mexican-Spiced Pork Chops*
- Green beans
- Roasted Brussels Sprouts with Balsamic Dressing.*
- Side salad, with Italian or oil and vinegar dressing
- Orange Jell-O cup, sugar-free
- Water infused with lime slices, and/or flavored gelatin without added sugar

Day 10

Breakfast

- 1–2 hard-boiled eggs
- Canadian bacon
- 4–6 ounces tomato juice, low-sodium

Midmorning Snack

- 1 The Laughing Cow Light Cheese Wedge
- Grape tomatoes

Lunch

- Sesame Chicken Salad.* Hint: If you are not at home for this meal, you should prepare it the night before.
- Pepper strips
- Strawberry Jell-O cup, sugar-free

Midafternoon Snack

- 4 ounces cottage cheese, reduced-fat or nonfat
- Celery sticks

Before-Dinner Snack (Optional)

- Raw veggies
- Hummus

Dinner

- No Crust Pizza*
- Hearty-sized salad. Hint: Add a variety of veggies such as cucumbers, carrots, tomatoes, red cabbage, pepper slices, mushrooms, etc. Top with Italian, oil and vinegar, or vinaigrette dressing.
- Black cherry Jell-O cup, artificially sweetened

Day 11

Breakfast

- Mini–Egg Beaters omelet. Spray microwave-safe dish or cup with cooking spray. Add ¼–½ cup Egg Beaters. Microwave on high for 1 minute. Stir, and cook an additional 15 seconds.
- 4–6 ounces diet cranberry juice

Midmorning Snack

- Peanut butter
- Carrot or celery sticks

Lunch

- Swiss cheese and roast beef roll-up. Hint: Add lettuce and other vegetables while rolling up.
- Baby carrots
- Italian coleslaw
- Strawberry Jell-O cup, sugar-free

Midafternoon Snack

- 1–2 Mini Babybel Light cheese wheels
- Grape tomatoes

Before-Dinner Snack (Optional)

- 10 peanuts in the shell (20 individual peanuts)

Dinner

- Asian Chicken Lettuce Wraps*
- Sautéed snow peas and broccoli slaw. Heat 1 teaspoon of canola or peanut oil in a medium skillet over medium-high heat. Add 1 package frozen (or 8 ounces fresh) snow peas and 1 cup broccoli slaw (also called confetti slaw). Sauté until softened, per your preference.
- Orange Jell-O cup, artificially sweetened

Day 12

Breakfast

- Scrambled eggs
- 1 ounce lean roast beef
- 4–6 ounces tomato juice, low-sodium

Midmorning Snack

- 4 ounces strawberry light yogurt, nonfat, artificially sweetened
- 10 cashews

Lunch

- 2–3 ham and Swiss roll-ups
- Italian coleslaw. Hint: If you are feeling adventurous, place the coleslaw inside the wraps.

- Sliced cucumbers
- Lime Jell-O cup, artificially sweetened

Midafternoon Snack

- 1–2 light string cheese sticks
- Celery sticks

Before-Dinner Snack (Optional)

- Pepper strips
- ¼ cup guacamole

Dinner

- Grilled Steak Salad*
- Grilled fresh asparagus
- Cherry Jell-O cup, artificially sweetened

Day 13

Breakfast

- Quick mini-omelet. Spray microwave-safe cup or dish with cooking spray. Add ½ cup Egg Beaters Florentine. Microwave on high for 1 minute. Stir, and heat for an additional 15 seconds.
- Diet cranberry juice

Midmorning Snack

- 1–2 The Laughing Cow Light Cheese Wedges
- Baby carrots

Lunch

- Large cheeseburger. Hint: Can be from a fast-food restaurant, but pitch the bun.

- Side salad. Hint: Cut up the burger and place it on top of the salad.
- Lime Jell-O cup, sugar-free

Midafternoon Snack

- Blueberry light yogurt, nonfat, artificially sweetened
- 20 walnuts

Before-Dinner Snack (Optional)

- 1–2 slices Swiss cheese, made from 2% milk
- 10 cashews

Dinner

- Sloppy joes, no bun
- Green beans
- Sliced tomatoes
- Coleslaw or side salad
- Cherry Jell-O cup, sugar-free

Day 14

Breakfast

- 1–2 hard-boiled eggs
- Canadian bacon
- 4–6 ounces tomato juice, low-sodium

Midmorning Snack

- 4 ounces strawberry-banana light yogurt
- 10 walnuts

Lunch

- Grilled chicken breast
- Sliced tomatoes
- Baby carrots
- Side salad, with dressing
- Raspberry Jell-O cup, sugar-free

Midafternoon Snack

- 1–2 light string cheese sticks
- Grape tomatoes

Before-Dinner Snack (Optional)

- 10 peanuts in the shell (20 individual peanuts)

Dinner

- Southwestern Blackened Chicken Salad.* Hint: This could also be a restaurant meal. Just ask them to hold the tortilla strips, and choose grilled chicken instead of crispy chicken. To prepare at home: Make a salad with crispy lettuce, tomatoes, pepper slices, sliced scallions, and avocado slices or guacamole, top with grilled chicken and a small handful of light shredded Colby-Jack cheese, and dress with ranch dressing. You could also add black beans (from a can, drained and rinsed).
- Orange Jell-O cup, sugar-free

CHAPTER 5

Phase Two: Take It Up a Notch!

You have made it through the first 14 days—congratulations! You are probably tired of eggs and really missing fruit. And you are thrilled with your weight loss progress. You can see that your stomach is much flatter and your clothes are much looser around your waist. Now it is time to get into Phase Two, which includes all the key DASH diet food. This is still going to be lower in starchy foods than you are probably used to, and will build on what you have learned in the initial 14 days. You will add back more dairy (or dairy substitutes), fruits, and whole grains to have a complete, balanced diet. And it will feel so easy, since you have made the foundation into a habit.

Phase Two: The DASH Solution

To introduce you to the complete weight loss solution, we, once again, give you our ultrasimple yet completely doable plan.

Below is an overview of the foods you will be incorporating into your diet during this next phase.

Quick Overview

Everyday Foods

- 2–3 servings low-fat protein-rich foods (lean meats, fish, poultry, beans, lentils, eggs, soy foods)
- 3–4 servings of low-fat or nonfat dairy (cheese, milk, yogurt)
- 4 or more servings of nonstarchy vegetables, and corn or peas
- 2–4 servings of fruit each day (no more than 4–6 ounces of juice)
- 1–2 servings nuts or seeds
- 1–2 servings whole grains, if desired

Remember to have some protein at each meal and snack.

Occasional Foods

- 3–4 servings refined, starchy, or sugary foods each week, maximum

This might be two pieces of pizza twice a month (fill up on salad to avoid overdoing), a smaller portion of dessert at a restaurant once a week, bread at a restaurant if it is really great. The point is to save your carbs for something really terrific, rather than wasting them on mediocre foods. I am not a proponent of low-carb breads or pasta. Save your carb calories for really special foods, and don't develop the habit of reintroducing unneeded breads or pasta. It is too easy to slip back into a carb-laden way of eating again. Black-and-white decisions about what to eat are much easier.

Include Moderate-Sized Servings of These Foods

Foods That Are Protein Rich and Low in Saturated Fat

- Lean meats, fish, and poultry
- Beans, lentils, soy foods
- Low-fat or nonfat cheeses
- Egg substitutes, egg whites, or whole eggs
- Nonfat milk and yogurt (with little or no added sugar). Yogurt should be less than 120 calories for an 8-ounce serving or less than 100 calories for a 6-ounce serving.

Heart-Healthy Fats

- Avocados, olives
- Vegetable oils, especially olive oil, canola oil, and nut oils. (Coconut oil and palm oil are excluded, since they are high in saturated fat.)
- Salad dressings, especially those based on the above oils. Some regular mayonnaise is okay, too.

Foods That Are Protein Rich and Contain Healthy Fat

- Nuts and seeds
- Fatty fish

Enjoy as Much of These Foods as You Want

- Sugar-free Jell-O
- Nonstarchy vegetables (exclusions include potatoes, winter squash, corn, etc.). Feel free to include carrots and tomatoes, which are often unnecessarily avoided in

lower-carb plans. Corn can be eaten during Phase Two, but not in unlimited quantities.

Foods to Limit

- Starchy foods (except beans) and sugary foods. This means very limited bread, pasta, potatoes, etc. Avoid foods fried in batter. Avoid rice cakes, pretzels, and similar foods.
- Some ketchup and BBQ sauce are okay.
- Foods with saturated, hydrogenated, or trans fats. These include most pastries, cookies, and snack crackers.
- Alcohol only in moderation. Moderate alcohol consumption is associated with lower risk of heart disease; however, alcohol is a source of empty calories. Replace one fruit serving with one 3½-ounce glass of wine.
- Caffeinated beverages other than with meals or snacks.
- Avoid foods that are high in saturated fats or that don't taste good. Don't start up your carb cravings by including lots of reduced-sugar pastries or cookies.

Guidelines

- Do not skip meals or afternoon snacks. This will keep your blood sugar steady, and help you avoid hunger. Relax after work, and have a before-dinner snack to avoid overeating.
- Thirty minutes or more of exercise is recommended each day. Aerobic exercise, such as walking, running, or biking, will burn extra calories and help lower blood sugar. Strength-building exercise increases the amount of calories that you burn all day long, and improves your ability to remove sugar from your blood. Your energy level should be higher than in the first phase.

- Get plenty of fluids, at least 8 glasses per day. (Yes, caffeinated beverages count, as does Jell-O.)
- Tell yourself that you have created a healthy way of eating that will become a habit.
- Focus on making your plate colorful. Salads should have more than just green lettuce. More fruits and vegetables make this a great way to eat.
- Focus on your weight loss results. Your success will keep you focused and make it easier to stay on track.
- Measure your waist circumference. If it starts to increase again, go back to the stricter plan to get refocused. Lower waist circumference is associated with improved health, and reflects a healthy plan.

Serving Sizes for the DASH Diet Weight Loss Solution

Typical serving sizes for the DASH diet are listed below. Larger men will need larger portion sizes of the protein-rich foods. Note: Serving sizes for a variety of foods (even those that you should strictly limit) are included in this list. It is not a list of recommended foods, just a relatively representative listing of serving sizes.

Grains, Starches, and Sugars

- 1 slice bread, ¼ bagel, ½ English muffin or hamburger or hot dog bun
- ½ cup cooked pasta, cereal (oatmeal, grits, wheat), corn, or potatoes
- ⅓ cup rice
- 1 ounce dry cereal (80–100 calories)

- 2 cups popcorn
- 2 small cookies

Fruits

- 4 ounces juice, or a small to medium fruit
- ¼ cup dried fruit
- ½ cup canned fruit
- 1 cup diced raw fruit

Vegetables

- ½ cup cooked vegetables
- 1 cup leafy greens
- 6 ounces vegetable juice

Dairy

- 8 ounces milk or 8 ounces yogurt
- 1 ounce cheese
- ½ cup cottage cheese

Beans, Nuts, Seeds

- ¼ cup beans
- ¼ cup nuts
- ¼ cup seeds

Cooked Lean Meat, Fish, Poultry, Eggs

- 3 ounces is about the size of the palm of a woman's hand
- 4 ounces is about the size of a woman's palm and thumb
- 5 ounces is about the size of a man's palm
- 1 egg = 1 ounce, 2 egg whites = 1 ounce

Fats, Fatty Sauces

- 1 tablespoon salad dressing
- 1 teaspoon butter, oil

Phase Two Eating

Meal plans for Phase Two and beyond are included in Chapter 6, but I have added some meal suggestions below to help you in planning your new lifestyle. You can mix or match meals and snacks. However, avoid overdoing the grains (maximum of 3 servings per day), and be sure to get at least 3 servings of fruit, 5 servings of vegetables, and 2–3 servings of dairy per day.

Breakfasts

Protein-Rich Breakfasts

- Eggs or egg substitutes (may use some cheese 1–2 days)
- 1–2 slices Canadian bacon or ham (both are considered lean meats) or soy alternatives
- 4 ounces of juice, if desired
- Milk or yogurt
- If you don't like eggs, the lunchtime roll-ups make great breakfast meals.

Cereal Breakfasts

- Whole grain cereal (less than 5 grams sugar per serving). A serving is 1 ounce by weight (½ cup of cooked oatmeal) and should be less than 100 calories. Watch out for serving sizes on cereal!

- Milk, yogurt, or hot chocolate made with skim milk, cocoa powder, and sugar substitute
- 4 ounces of juice
- Fruit for sweetening the cereal

Midmorning Snacks

Have 1–2 of the following (include some protein):

- Low-fat cheese, such as The Laughing Cow Light Wedges, Mini Babybel Light, light string cheese, or light cottage cheese (4-ounce size)
- Veggies, including celery, radishes, carrots, cucumbers, sliced peppers, grape or cherry tomatoes
- 4–6 ounces yogurt, unsweetened or artificially sweetened
- 1 serving fruit
- Nuts—¼ cup or less, which is about 20 nuts. (If having nuts and cheese, limit to 10 nuts.)

Lunches

- Salad with lots of types of veggies topped with a good protein source, with dressing, without croutons, occasionally with regular cheese, preferably with light cheese, *or*
- Egg salad, egg white salad, chicken salad, and/or tuna salad, *or*
- Roll-ups made with low-fat cheese and ham, turkey, or lean roast beef

And some of the following:

- Veggies and/or side salad with dressing
- 1 serving of fruit

- 4–6 ounces yogurt (unsweetened or artificially sweetened) or 8 ounces milk
- 10–20 nuts
- Sugar-free Jell-O

Midafternoon Snacks (and add a before-dinner snack, if desired)

Same as the morning snacks. Additional choices include:

- Pepper strips dipped in ¼ cup guacamole, hummus, or salad dressing
- 10 peanuts in the shell (20 individual peanuts)

Dinners

- Lean meat, fish, or poultry
- Nonstarchy veggies (top with reduced-fat cheese if desired)
- Salad with dressing
- Milk, if desired

If you are craving pasta, have pasta sauce (meaty or with beans—you want the protein) on top of veggies. Top with cheese, and brown under the broiler in an ovenproof dish. Or use spaghetti squash as your pasta replacement. You can follow our recipe for Meaty Sauce over Spaghetti Squash.*

Make a "pizza" with pizza sauce and ground beef, no crust, top with veggies and reduced-fat mozzarella, and bake until the cheese is melted. See the recipe for No Crust Pizza.*

Desserts Could Include

- Sugar-free Jell-O
- 1 serving of fruit

- Frozen bars with less than 100 calories, and no added sugar. (Example: Healthy Choice Fudge Bars.) Avoid higher-fat and higher-calorie desserts.

Dining Out Meals

Breakfasts

- Eggs, omelets, oatmeal or other whole grain cereal (watch out for grain portion sizes, limit cereals to 1 serving, which is ½ cup cooked cereals)
- Some bacon or lean breakfast meat is okay
- 1 serving of fruit and/or tomatoes
- 4 ounces juice
- 8 ounces milk or 4–6 ounces unsweetened yogurt

Hint: Instead of toast or potatoes, have fruit and/or veggies.

Lunches

- Salads topped with a good protein source
- Burger or grilled chicken without the bun, and with side vegetables and/or salad or coleslaw
- Skim milk or yogurt, if available

Hint: Almost every fast-food restaurant, supermarket, or convenience store has great salads now.

Dinners

- Lean meat, fish, or poultry
- Side vegetables. In Italian restaurants, ask if they will substitute veggies for pasta.

- Side salad with dressing
- Small amount of dessert, if it is really, really good, and only if you are still hungry

Hit the Grocery Store to Stock Up On...

- Egg Beaters or other egg substitutes, with or without vegetables
- Eggs
- Individually packaged light cheeses such as: The Laughing Cow Light Wedges, Mini Babybel Light, light string cheese, light cottage cheese (4-ounce size), and Kraft 2% singles
- Sugar-free Jell-O
- Skim milk
- Nonfat yogurt with little or no sugar. Less than 120 calories for 8 ounces, or 100 calories for 6 ounces. You can also find six-packs of 4-ounce sizes (less than 60 calories) for snacks.
- Lean meats, fish, and poultry, or beans and soy foods for vegetarian meals. Lean meats include 90% or 95% lean ground beef, ground turkey with only white meat (no fat or skin), beef or pork tenderloin, beef or pork loin chops, sirloin, New York strip steaks, all round cuts, chuck cuts. Select is the leanest grade of beef.
- Sliced light cheese and lean deli meats
- Bagged fresh cut-up veggies, such as lettuce, carrots, broccoli, broccoli slaw, and cabbage slaw
- Frozen veggies; frozen fruits, if you like them
- Unsweetened applesauce
- Great fresh fruits

- Olive oil and/or canola oil. Salad dressings containing these oils, if possible.
- Egg salad, tuna salad, and chicken salad
- Salad bar for cut-up fresh fruits and veggies, such as peppers, cucumbers, radishes, celery, and more, for salads and snacks
- Nuts in the shell. Choose nuts that are not addictive for you. Shelling nuts slows you down, to help you avoid overeating them.
- Guacamole and/or hummus

Avoid foods that are high in saturated fats or that don't taste good.

Plan, Plan, Plan

- Take your lunches and snacks to work if you can't find the right foods in your cafeteria or at the restaurants you frequent. Either stock your minifridge at the office or bring an insulated bag with all the right foods.
- Make sure you keep all the right foods on hand.
- Do not skip meals or afternoon snacks.
- Plan what you will eat for each meal and snack, each day.
- Plan what you will eat *before* you go to a restaurant.
- Don't fill up your diet with synthetic low-carb foods. Focus on healthy, real foods.
- Remember your goal. Then plan to succeed.

Overview of Phase Two Diet Patterns

The following table will help you understand the food group patterns for the DASH Diet Weight Loss Solution, Phase Two.

Phase Two Food Group Servings Per Day

	Smaller appetite	Moderate appetite	Larger appetite
Nonstarchy vegetables	Unlimited		
Dairy	2–3	2–3	3–4
Nuts, beans, seeds	1–2	1–3	2–4
Lean meat, fish, poultry, eggs	5–6 ounces	6–8 ounces	8–11 ounces
Fats	1–2	2–3	3–4
Whole Grains	2–3	2–3	2–4
Fruit	2–3	2–4	3–5
Refined grains, sweets	Rarely, 2–3 times per week		

You have created a foundation for a lifetime of healthy eating. You have learned to fill your plate with lots of colorful vegetables; you are choosing lean meats, fish, and poultry and other low-fat protein-rich foods; and you have added low-fat dairy to your regimen. Fruits, yogurt, veggies, and nuts make great snacks. What a great start to a plan that will improve your health, help you reach and maintain your weight goal, and be easy to follow!

Meeting the Challenges

How I met the challenges from Phase One: _____

_____

Challenges expected with the complete DASH plan: _____

_____

_____

How I will overcome these challenges: _____

_____

CHAPTER 6

Your Plate Overflows! An Abundance of DASH Diet Menus for Weight Loss

New menus! And more choices! We bring back fruit, milk, whole wheat bread and cereals, not to mention, additional dessert ideas. However, you will still be avoiding starchy, refined foods and foods with added sugars.

You will have more choices for beverages, including lattes, milk, and hot chocolate. Other than these dairy-containing drinks and juices, we have not specified any other beverages so you are free to choose any that you like, continuing to avoid sugar. Go easy on reintroducing alcohol, since it can reduce your resolve regarding the diet plan.

And again, you can mix or match meals and snacks. Just try to avoid going over 3 servings of whole grains per day, and make sure you get 2–3 servings of dairy, at least 3 servings of fruit, and 5 servings of vegetables.

You can continue to have virtually unlimited sugar-free Jell-O. And another favorite treat is a Healthy Choice Premium Fudge Bar. These have no added sugar, are very low in fat, and less than 100 calories, but you would never know that they were anything but real ice cream.

Our use of brand names does not imply any endorsement of these brands. They are used just because they are easily identifiable. Any similar foods with approximately the same calories and nutritional profile will be great as well.

Day 1

Breakfast

- ¾ cup Wheaties (1 ounce by weight)
- 8 ounces skim milk
- 4–6 ounces strawberries or raspberries

Midmorning Snack (Optional)

- 1–2 The Laughing Cow Light Cheese Wedges
- Grape tomatoes

Lunch

- 2–3 turkey and Swiss roll-ups
- Baby carrots
- Small plum

Midafternoon Snack

- 6 ounces blueberry light yogurt
- 10 cashews

Before-Dinner Snack (Optional)

- 10 peanuts in the shell (20 individual peanuts)

Dinner

- Pan-seared tilapia. Heat 1 tablespoon olive oil in a skillet over medium-high heat. Cook about 4 minutes per side, or until the fish flakes easily with a fork. Before finishing, place about 1 pat of butter or margarine in the pan, and allow the melted butter to coat all the pieces. (To serve four, choose four 4-ounce tilapia filets.)
- Mango-Melon Salsa*
- Fresh asparagus
- Strawberry Jell-O cup, sugar-free

Day 2

Breakfast

- Hot chocolate. To 8 ounces skim milk, add 1 heaping teaspoon unsweetened cocoa and 2 packets Splenda or Truvia.
- 1–2 hard-boiled eggs
- 6–8 ounces light cranberry juice. Hint: Light cranberry juice has more calories than the diet version, but you may prefer it.
- 4–6 ounces strawberries

Midmorning Snack (Optional)

- 6 ounces key lime light yogurt, nonfat, artificially sweetened
- 10 ounces almonds

Lunch

- Turkey and Swiss sandwich. Put 2–4 ounces turkey and a slice of reduced-fat Swiss cheese on two pieces light whole wheat bread; add lettuce, tomato, and any other veggies or condiments that you choose.

- Pepper strips
- Coleslaw or side salad
- Raspberry Jell-O cup, artificially sweetened

Midafternoon Snack

- 1 clementine orange
- 1–2 The Laughing Cow Light Cheese Wedges

Before-Dinner Snack (Optional)

- Pepper strips
- ¼–½ cup hummus

Dinner

- Meaty Sauce over Spaghetti Squash*
- Side salad, with Italian, oil and vinegar, or vinaigrette dressing
- Healthy Choice Premium Fudge Bar

Day 3

Breakfast

- ½ cup oatmeal, cooked: topped with cinnamon, Splenda Brown Sugar Blend, or Truvia, and 1 tablespoon chopped almonds (optional)
- ½ banana, medium or large
- 4–6 ounces tomato juice, low-sodium
- Latte: 8 ounces skim milk, 2 ounces espresso

Midmorning Snack (Optional)

- 1 stick light cheese
- Baby carrots

Lunch

- Acapulco Tuna Salad* in ½ whole wheat pita pocket. Hint: Feel free to add other veggies, such as lettuce, tomatoes, red cabbage, and grated carrots.
- Sliced bell peppers
- Orange Jell-O cup, artificially sweetened

Midafternoon Snack

- 4–6 ounces strawberries
- 10 cashews

Before-Dinner Snack (Optional)

- 10 peanuts in the shell (20 individual peanuts)

Dinner

- Naked Chicken Piccata*
- Green beans
- Sliced tomatoes
- Side salad, with Italian dressing
- 4–6 ounces raspberries on ½–1 cup frozen yogurt, non-fat, artificially sweetened

Day 4

Breakfast

- 1–3 scrambled eggs
- 1 slice whole wheat toast (light, if desired)
- 1 tablespoon jelly or jam
- 4–6 ounces orange juice
- Latte or 8 ounces skim milk

Midmorning Snack (Optional)

- 4–6 ounces blueberries
- 10 almonds

Lunch

- 2–3 Muenster cheese and roast beef roll-ups. Hint: Accessorize per your taste. You could add lettuce for the wrap and stuff with grated carrots or red cabbage in the center.
- Italian coleslaw. Hint: This is regular coleslaw with thin pepper strips, grated carrots, and an oil and vinegar dressing.
- Small peach

Midafternoon Snack

- 6 ounces strawberry light yogurt, nonfat, artificially sweetened

Before-Dinner Snack (Optional)

- Baby carrots dipped in 2 tablespoons peanut butter

Dinner

- Zucchini Lasagna*
- Side salad: lettuce, grape tomatoes, red cabbage, and blue cheese crumbles or small slice of goat cheese, with oil and vinegar or vinaigrette dressing.
- Healthy Choice Premium Fudge Bar or other low-calorie, low-sugar, low-fat ice cream bar

Day 5

Breakfast

- Hot chocolate. To 8 ounces skim milk, add 1 heaping teaspoon unsweetened cocoa and 2 packets Splenda or Truvia.
- 1 cup raisin bran with 4 ounces skim milk
- 4–6 ounces orange-tangerine juice. Hint: You can substitute any kind of high-potassium juice that you like.

Midmorning Snack (Optional)

- 6 ounces blueberry light yogurt, nonfat, artificially sweetened

Lunch

- Peanut butter and jelly sandwich on whole wheat. Hint: Use light bread (about 45 calories per slice) and natural peanut butter. Hint: Natural peanut butter is unprocessed, meaning no hydrogenation or trans fats. It must be stored in the refrigerator after opening. Don't bother with the reduced-fat version, since the calories are identical. And the peanut butter fats are heart healthy. Before opening, we store upside down, to get some of the oil from the top better distributed throughout. Then on opening, mix well. The better the mixing, the less likely it is to be very hard when you get to the bottom. And if it is, put a portion in the microwave for about 10 seconds, to soften.
- Baby carrots
- Side salad with dressing (optional)
- Medium apple

Midafternoon Snack

- Grape tomatoes
- 1–2 light string cheese sticks

Before-Dinner Snack (Optional)

- Raw veggies
- ¼ cup guacamole

Dinner

- Chicken Souvlaki*
- ⅓ cup brown rice
- Greek salad. Chopped romaine lettuce hearts, diced cucumber, diced tomatoes, thinly sliced sweet red onions, feta cheese crumbles (if desired), and oil and vinegar or Italian dressing.
- Raspberry Jell-O cup, artificially sweetened

Day 6

Breakfast

- 8–12 ounces latte
- 1–3-egg veggie omelet
- 2–3 slices bacon
- 4–6 ounces tomato juice, low-sodium

Midmorning Snack (Optional)

- 4–6 ounces strawberries
- 10 cashews

Lunch

- Cheeseburger, with whole-wheat bun, if available. If not, have it without the bun.
- Broccoli
- Coleslaw
- Small or medium pear

Midafternoon Snack

- 2 deviled eggs
- Small or medium plum

Before-Dinner Snack (Optional)

- 10 peanuts in the shell (20 individual peanuts)

Dinner

- Blackened Chicken and Berry Salad*
- Healthy Choice Premium Fudge Bar or bar with similar nutritional properties

Hint: Think the dinner looks skimpy? Think again—this is a very high-flavor, complete, and satisfying meal.

Day 7

Breakfast

- ¾ cup Grape Nut Flakes. Hint: If you choose to substitute Grape Nuts, the serving size is ¼ cup to provide equal calories.
- ½ banana
- 8 ounces skim milk
- 4–6 ounces orange juice

Midmorning Snack (Optional)

- 1–2 The Laughing Cow Light Cheese Wedges
- Baby carrots

Lunch

- 1–2 vegetarian hot dogs, each on a slice of light whole wheat bread or whole wheat tortilla, with the condiments of your choice
- Sliced cucumbers
- Sliced tomatoes
- Italian coleslaw
- Lime Jell-O cup, sugar-free

Midafternoon Snack

- 6 ounces lemon light yogurt, nonfat, artificially sweetened
- 10 almonds

Before-Dinner Snack (Optional)

- Raw veggies
- ¼–½ cup hummus

Dinner

- Super-Easy, Lip-Smacking-Good Roasted Chicken and Winter Vegetables*
- Side salad, with Italian, oil and vinegar, or vinaigrette dressing
- 4–6 ounces raspberries on ½–1 cup frozen yogurt, nonfat, artificially sweetened

Hint: Your dinner veggies come from the chicken recipe. This is a great one-pot meal.

Day 8

Breakfast

- 1 whole-grain blueberry waffle, topped with blueberry jam
- 1–2 hard-boiled eggs
- Hot chocolate. To 8 ounces skim milk, add 1 heaping teaspoon unsweetened cocoa and 2 packets Splenda or Truvia.

Midmorning Snack (Optional)

- 4–6 ounces orange light yogurt, nonfat, artificially sweetened
- 10 walnuts

Lunch

- Sesame Chicken Salad.* Hint: This is definitely a make-ahead meal, but it's a great salad to have for several days.
- 1–1½ cups cherries

Midafternoon Snack

- Baby carrots
- 2 tablespoons peanut butter

Before-Dinner Snack (Optional)

- 1 slice Swiss cheese, made with 2% milk
- 6 Triscuit Hint of Salt crackers

Dinner

- The Frittata That Makes a Meal*
- Side salad

- Healthy Choice Premium Fudge Bar or other bar with similar nutritional properties

Day 9

Breakfast

- ½ cup cooked oatmeal, topped with cinnamon and Splenda Brown Sugar Blend or Truvia
- 8–12 ounces latte
- ½ medium banana
- 4–6 ounces light cranberry juice

Midmorning Snack

- 6 ounces strawberry-banana light yogurt, nonfat, artificially sweetened
- Baby carrots

Lunch

- Tuna salad in ½ whole grain pita. Hint: Stuff with lettuce, tomatoes, cabbage, and/or other veggies.
- Cucumber slices
- Side salad with dressing
- Small or medium plum

Midafternoon Snack

- 1–2 string cheese sticks
- Grape tomatoes

Before-Dinner Snack (Optional)

- 10 peanuts in the shell (20 individual peanuts)

Dinner

- The World's Best Meatloaf*
- Creamy Cauliflower Mashed Potatoes*
- ½ cup sweet corn
- 1 tablespoon catsup or barbecue sauce, if desired

Hint: The meatloaf provides meals for several days, which makes this a great dish, especially on weekends.

Day 10

Breakfast

- 1–2 hard-boiled eggs
- 4–6 ounces strawberries
- 8–12 ounces latte or hot chocolate
- 4–6 ounces orange juice

Midmorning Snack (Optional)

- 1–2 The Laughing Cow Light Cheese Wedges
- Grape tomatoes

Lunch

- Ham and swiss on light whole wheat bread, topped with lettuce and any other desired veggies
- Sliced tomatoes
- Italian coleslaw
- 2 slices fresh pineapple

Midafternoon Snack

- 6 ounces banana light yogurt, nonfat, artificially sweetened
- 10 almonds

Before-Dinner Snack (Optional)

- Raw veggies
- ¼ cup guacamole

Dinner

- Mango-Berry Salsa with Grilled Pork Loin*
- Roasted Brussels Sprouts with Balsamic Dressing*
- Healthy Choice Premium Fudge Bar or other bar with similar nutritional properties

Day 11

Breakfast

- 1 shredded wheat biscuit
- 8 ounces skim milk
- 4–6 ounces strawberries
- 4–6 ounces orange juice

Midmorning Snack (Optional)

- 6 ounces lemon light yogurt, nonfat, artificially sweetened
- Baby carrots

Lunch

- Poached Chicken Salad with Grapes and Walnuts*

Midafternoon Snack

- Small or medium peach
- 10 cashews

Before-Dinner Snack (Optional)

- 1–2 slices Swiss cheese, made from 2% milk

Dinner

- Alaska Walnut-Crusted Salmon with Raspberry Coulis*
- Glazed Carrots*
- Side salad with dressing
- 4–6 ounces raspberries on ½–1 cup frozen yogurt, non-fat, artificially sweetened

Day 12

Breakfast

- Mini–Egg Beaters Southwestern Style omelet. Spray microwave-safe dish or cup with cooking spray. Add ¼–½ cup Egg Beaters Southwestern Style. Microwave on high for 1 minute. Stir, and cook an additional 15 seconds.
- 1 slice whole wheat toast, topped with jam or jelly
- Cantaloupe wedge
- 4–6 ounces orange juice

Midmorning Snack (Optional)

- 1–2 The Laughing Cow Light Cheese Wedges
- Grape tomatoes

Lunch

- Tuna salad sandwich, on 2 slices light whole wheat bread, topped with tomato slices, lettuce, and any additional vegetables you like
- Sliced radishes
- 4 ounces tomato soup, reduced-sodium
- Small apple

Midafternoon Snack

- 4–6 ounces strawberry-banana light yogurt, nonfat, artificially sweetened
- 10 cashews

Before-Dinner Snack (Optional)

- Raw veggies
- ¼–½ cup hummus

Dinner

- Blackened Chicken with Avocado-Papaya Salsa*
- 1 cup petite sweet peas
- Side salad with dressing
- 4–6 ounces strawberries on ½–1 cup frozen yogurt, nonfat, artificially sweetened

Day 13

Breakfast

- 1 cup Cheerios
- ½ sliced medium banana
- 8 ounces skim milk
- 4–6 ounces orange juice

Midmorning Snack (Optional)

- 6 ounces strawberry light yogurt, nonfat, artificially sweetened
- 10 walnuts

Lunch

- 1–2 Turkey Roll-ups with Blueberry Salsa*
- Side salad with dressing
- 1 clementine orange

Midafternoon Snack

- 1–2 light string cheese sticks
- Baby carrots

Before-Dinner Snack (Optional)

- 10 peanuts in the shell (20 individual peanuts)

Dinner

- Baked halibut. On a baking sheet covered with olive oil cooking spray, place the halibut steaks. Sprinkle with herbs (your choice, or lemon-pepper seasoning mix) and top with a lemon slice. Drizzle with olive oil (or spray again). Bake in a preheated 450°F oven for 14 minutes or until fish is no longer translucent and flakes with a fork.
- Roasted Broccoli, Cauliflower, and Carrots*
- Romaine and Blood Orange Salad*
- Healthy Choice Premium Fudge Bar, or other bar with similar nutritional properties

Day 14

Breakfast

- 1–2 hard-boiled eggs
- ½ whole grain English muffin, topped with butter or margarine

- 8–12 ounces latte
- 4–6 ounces strawberries
- 4–6 ounces tomato juice, low-sodium

Midmorning Snack (Optional)

- 1–2 light string cheese sticks
- Grape tomatoes

Lunch

- Grilled chicken sandwich on light whole wheat bread
- Tomato slices
- Cucumber slices
- Italian coleslaw
- Small plum

Midafternoon Snack

- 6 ounces raspberry light yogurt, nonfat, artificially sweetened
- 10 walnuts

Before-Dinner Snack (Optional)

- Pepper strips
- Black bean salsa

Dinner

- Mexican Meatloaf*
- Mashed Sweet Potatoes with Maple and Orange*
- Green Beans and Peppers*
- 4–6 ounces mixed fresh berries

CHAPTER 7

Move It to Lose It with DASH

The second most obvious component of any weight loss plan is exercise. Many of you may be groaning and saying that you hate to exercise, but a little physical activity can go a long way toward helping you feel younger and look better. I'm not talking about spending hours on the treadmill every day of the week or training for a marathon. You can be more active, burn more calories, and get fit by making small changes in your lifestyle—and doing things you enjoy.

Consider this: In addition to improving health, activity also makes you feel younger. It is one of the ways that you actually can turn back the clock. When you start to exercise, within the first month, you will have a much higher energy level. You will have more bounce in your step. Exercise has long been known to be associated with lower rates of depression and can relieve stress. And now research shows that exercise is associated with increased brain volume and slower age-related deterioration of cognitive abilities.

What is it going to take to find the motivation to start exercising? Perhaps you can change from the "e-word" to an "a-word," and look for ways to increase your *activity* level. Too many of us are very sedentary at work, stuck behind a computer screen all day. Then we drive home, pick up some food on the way, and eat in front of the TV screen. If you think about how to be more physically active, you could increase your calorie burning very easily several times during any given day. What if you park a little farther from your office? Then walk around the office or workplace a few times before you go to your desk. If there are some stairs, use them. Instead of sending an e-mail to your colleague, get up and go talk to her face-to-face. Walk for five minutes before and after lunch. Take an afternoon walk break before you have your snack. At the end of the day, go to the grocery store to buy food that you will make for dinner. You will be more active simply by standing up while making dinner. After dinner, stand up, and walk in place or on a treadmill for a few minutes. Or better yet, go outside for a walk.

That was all so easy. It's so simple to add little bits of activity to your day. It is especially important to find things that are fun for you. If you are very social, then exercising or walking with a friend will be something you are more likely to continue. Team and competitive sports appeal to many people. If your schedule is very hectic, you may want an exercise that you can do at home, to minimize changing and transit time. If you really hate to exercise, having a personal trainer with scheduled appointments may be what is needed to stay on track. If you are already physically active, trying something new may be the ticket to boosting your metabolism.

When you think about the kinds of activities you should be doing, consider cardio or aerobic activity as the first line of defense against weight creep, heart disease, diabetes, hypertension, and all those other bad things. You want to do some kind of aerobic activity most days of the week. Next should be some kind of strength exercise. I cannot emphasize enough how much benefit you will get from that type of exercise. By toning and firming your muscles, you will literally make your body feel and look much younger. Once or twice a week should be enough. You may also find benefit from balance and flexibility exercises such as yoga or tai chi, which you can do several times per week, or even daily.

Your goal should be to do something most days of the week. If you try to exercise every day, you are likely to hit at least five days a week. However, if you plan to exercise five days a week, you are likely to hit only three days, and pretty soon, you are maybe exercising one day a week. Once you have started to exercise on a regular basis, think about how much time you are devoting to activity. If you are trying to lose weight, most people need 60 minutes of activity each day. Once you get to the maintenance phase, 30 minutes daily should be good. Unless you want to do more. (Yay!)

Walking, jogging, or running require very little equipment and are very low-cost. You can even walk in place in front of your TV if it isn't safe outside or the weather isn't good enough. Get a pedometer to track your steps. To be healthy, it is recommended that most people take 10,000 steps per day. You may be shocked at how low your number is. But everyone starts somewhere, and you can slowly increase your numbers to bring them closer to the 10,000 steps goal. Walking around the office, the neighborhood, or even at home is an easy way to get started. Remember that sitting all day really slows down your metabolism, making it more of a challenge to get any benefit out of small amounts of exercise. So start to make your entire day more active, to get more of a payoff.

For strength exercises, you can go to a gym or use small weights or bands at home. I have used and often recommend the strength exercises that you will find in the Strong Women series of books by Miriam Nelson, PhD. Pilates can also improve strength and can be done at home with videos or in classes at your local park district or gym.

If you have mobility problems, try chair exercising. Put on some music, and move and groove in your seat. There was a recent news article about a woman with knee problems who went to a Zumba class and did all the movements while seated. She lost 70 pounds in a year. By that time, her joints didn't hurt as much, and she was able to do more activity, which further propelled her weight loss. But you don't have to go to a class. You could watch a video or do Zumba with a DVD or video game. Water exercise can also be great for people with mobility problems. Many hospitals have health centers with "arthritis pools," which are much warmer and make movement much easier.

Video games now can actually help you become more active while at home and fit into your own schedule. Of course, videos or walking or running podcasts can also be great ways to add some focus to your workout routines. If you love music, make your own playlist or listen to your favorite station while you walk, run, and move. Dancing feels more like fun, and can help you really get physically active either in the privacy of your own home, at a class, or out at a club.

Do you already have home exercise equipment? Treadmills, ellipticals, or stationary bikes are wonderful for aerobic activity. Make the experience less boring by listening to your favorite music, watching TV or a movie, listening to talk radio, or listening to an audiobook. Exercise that you can do at home is more likely to get done.

Lots of people like to engage in physical activity with friends. They think of it as play. They play golf, basketball, soccer, football, volleyball, tennis, or go bowling. Get your best friend to join you for classes at the gym, go for a walk, go Rollerblading, go hiking, or train for a 5K. If you have a supportive significant other, go out dancing or take dancing lessons. The point is, if you do something that is fun or feels like play, you will be more likely to continue the activity.

Need to grease the skids? Get the right exercise shoes, clothes, and equipment if needed. Try to remove any barriers to exercise. If you don't have the right gear, then go out and buy it (within your budget). Then lay out the clothes and gear the night before. You know the obstacles that are going to get in the way of exercising more. You are the only one who can set the stage for success.

The timing of your exercise matters, too. No, you don't increase the fat burning by choosing the right time of day. But you are less likely to skip exercise that is scheduled in the morning as compared to later in the day, when life tends to intervene. If you have to be a chauffeur most afternoons, that is not going to work for a regular exercise time (unless your exercise is walking back and forth on the soccer sidelines— which works on all counts). Or if you often have errands that you need to do after work or you have to work late, you will be tempted to skip "just this once." The flip side of this advice would be to schedule your home exercise time for something that you do every evening. If you always watch TV at 8:00 p.m., get on your treadmill or walk in place while you watch. Being realistic about your schedule will make the exercise component more likely to happen.

And to have positive reinforcement for developing your exercise habit, use our tracking form to keep a record of your activities. If you can see how your actions are building up, you will start to think of yourself a little differently. You are the one who is being successful at planning and reaching your goals. So decide that you *will* exercise.

1. Plan which types of exercise, activity, and play you will do.
2. Decide what time will work best for your schedule.
3. If you need others, identify the people and ensure that your schedules all align.
4. Get the gear, buy the game, or make the playlist.
5. Plan for more routine activity during your day.

My Actions to Add More Activity to My Days

Buy gym shoes _____   Buy gear _____

Identify the times _____ and days _____

Identify barriers to activity _____

Plans to remove the barriers _____

PART II

The Secrets of the DASH Diet Foods

CHAPTER 8

High-Carb, Low-Carb, What Should We Do?

Back in the late 1980s and the 1990s, high-grain diets were encouraged. People really went overboard with this philosophy; remember the huge plates of pasta and bottomless bread baskets? And Americans became fatter. Who could burn off all those calories if you weren't training for marathons all the time?

All those carb-loaded meals really wreaked havoc with people's health as well. We are currently in an epidemic of diabetes and insulin resistance (an inability to respond well to insulin), which can have many bad health consequences. And for people with insulin resistance, the high intake of starch from the grains eventually wears out the ability of the body to produce enough insulin to keep blood sugar under control, which can lead to diabetes. The bottom line: If you are struggling with your weight, and especially if you carry your extra weight around your waist, it is very important to avoid excess starch and sugar.

Regardless of weight or health issues, when you choose carbs, you would like them to be great sources of fiber, vitamins, minerals, and other important plant nutrients, while being relatively low in calories. Preferably, you will go easy on the carbs that are mostly refined, empty-calorie foods and/or are high in saturated and trans fats.

Fruits and Vegetables

Fruits and vegetables fit the bill for highly desirable carbs. They are two of the key food groups for the DASH Diet Weight Loss Solution. They are rich in vitamins, minerals, fiber, and antioxidants. By weight, they are mostly water, so the calories are low, but they are very filling. Fruits and vegetables are rich in the plant compounds known as phytochemicals (*phyto-* means "plant"). These chemicals include antioxidants and the compounds that produce color, scents, and flavor. Most of the "superfoods" are fruits and vegetables. However, it is more important to have a healthy diet than to just focus on trying to include a few of the healthiest fruits and vegetables into your regular diet. "Eat the rainbow" is an easy way to think about healthy eating. The more color on your plate, the more healthful it is likely to be. And the more variety in your diet, the better.

While research has shown that vegetable juice can help with successful weight loss on the DASH diet, in general you would like your fruits and vegetables to be whole. You want the fiber. You want the bulk of whole foods. You want the meal to keep you feeling full longer than 30 minutes. This is especially important to remember with fruit juices; try to limit them to 4 to 6 ounces per day. It's better to have whole fruits.

Whole Grains

When we have grains, we want them to be whole grains. Fiber, phytochemicals, vitamins, and minerals from whole grains are very good. Studies have shown that people who have more whole grains in their diets tend to be less likely to develop diabetes.

For people with sensitivity to gluten, it is absolutely fine to substitute gluten-free (GF) whole grains for wheat products. (For more information on food sensitivities or allergies, see Appendix A.) With the DASH Diet Weight Loss Solution, it actually will be easier to follow a GF plan. Most foods are made without any hidden additives and little flour is used in food preparation, so what you see is what you eat. Cutting out any gluten foods can explain why people often feel so much better during the first two weeks, when no grains are included in the plan.

When choosing cereals and breads, the only flour used in the food should be whole grain. The food manufacturers use lots of tricks to confuse us. For example, some cereal producers are putting small amounts of whole grains into their products, and then blazing the words "Whole Grain" across the front of the box. Surprisingly, you can't always use color to judge if a bread is whole grain. It might have caramel food coloring added to make it appear to be whole grain. When you are choosing cereals, try to get those with no more than 5 grams of sugar, and less than 250 milligrams of sodium.

Fiber

While many of us get too many calories each day, most of us get far too little of the fiber that we need. Recommendations are that we should get 14 grams per every 1,000 calories in our diet. This will not be a problem with the DASH diet, since your foundation will be vegetables, along with sufficient fruit, whole grains, and nuts, seeds, and beans. Just make sure you are getting 6 to 8 glasses of fluid each day. (Fiber without sufficient fluid can be constipating.) If you have trouble digesting the high-fiber foods, consider Beano to help avoid gas.

There are two main types of fiber—soluble and insoluble. Whole grains are especially rich in insoluble fiber, which is also referred to as roughage and helps to keep your bowel movements regular. Soluble fiber is found in large amounts in beans and fruits, and can help lower cholesterol by reducing the amount of dietary fats you absorb. It can also be beneficial for blood sugar control, since it slows the absorption of glucose during digestion. Regularity is enhanced, since it makes stools softer, bulkier, and easier to move through the intestines.

Research has shown that taking one type of soluble fiber, psyllium, at about 10 to 12 grams per day, can reduce cholesterol by about 3% to 14%. If you decide to add psyllium to your daily regimen, increase the dosage slowly until you reach the 10-to-12-gram target. (Check the package for serving sizes.) Be sure to drink plenty of fluids.

Not all soluble fiber helps to lower cholesterol. Another term for the ones that do is functional fiber, which helps to differentiate it from the soluble fiber that doesn't have this special health benefit. Several food manufacturers have introduced new soluble fiber products that have not been shown to have any health benefits, so choose proven products.

Examples of functional fiber include most of the naturally occurring plant fibers, including beta-glucan from oats, pectin in many types of fruit, psyllium fiber, and guar gum. For a list of specific foods rich in soluble fiber, see the table on page 97.

Some Good Sources of Fiber

	Soluble fiber, grams	Total fiber, grams
Apple, unpeeled	0.4	3.0
Pear, unpeeled	0.7	4.6
Raspberries, ½ cup	0.3	2.6
Prunes, 5	1.1	3.1
Avocado, ½	1.2	3.1
Sweet potato, ½ cup	0.5	1.9
Broccoli, 2 stalks	0.2	1.8
Carrots, ½ cup	0.4	1.9
Spaghetti sauce, ½ cup	0.6	3.0
Kidney beans, ½ cup	1.0	4.5
All-Bran cereal, ⅓ cup	0.7	8.1
Oatmeal, ¾ cup	1.2	2.7

Sugar Alcohols

Sugar alcohols, such as sorbitol and mannitol, have been long used as low-calorie sweeteners in foods. Even though they technically have the same calories as other carbohydrates, they are very difficult for the body to digest, which significantly reduces their caloric contribution to the diet. However, they can have one disturbing side effect if overconsumed. The sugar alcohols are well known to cause diarrhea. This can be especially noticeable in sugar-free baked goods, where they can be used in high amounts. And it can be especially problematic for someone who is taking metformin, a common diabetes medication, which also tends to increase the risk for diarrhea.

One strong benefit of the sugar alcohols is that they are noncariogenic, that is, they do not cause cavities and may prevent them and reduce the risk of periodontal disease. These products have been popular in sugar-free chewing gum for this reason.

Artificial Sweeteners

I was counseling a woman who had just had a heart attack two days prior. She had poorly controlled type 2 diabetes, which is often associated with increased risk for heart disease. She told me that her daughter wanted her to manage her disease more naturally, saying that artificial sweeteners were poison. Stunned, I explained that for her, with poor glucose control, the starchy foods and sugars were more likely to be poison. (Yes, I know the dietitians are cringing now, but the relatively young woman had just had a five-way bypass after her heart attack!)

Without enough insulin being produced by her body, sugar and starch would cause her blood sugar levels to rise, causing damage to her eyes, kidneys, nerves, and the lining of the veins and arteries. They would also cause her liver to become infiltrated with fat, and pump out excess triglycerides, further aggravating coronary artery disease. They would lower HDL levels (good cholesterol), which helps to keep arteries clean of cholesterol plaque buildup.

While it has been popular to denigrate artificial sweeteners, they do have a place in the diet for those people who want to have sweet-flavored foods but who can't handle the calories and/or sugar. Artificially sweetened dairy foods can be a great way to get the flavor without adding extra calories. However, artificially sweetened baked goods and pastries are still high in starch and usually have calories equal to the original foods. And for diabetics, since the starch breaks down to glucose during digestion, they are not a better choice than the regular baked goods with sugar. Furthermore, they are usually high in saturated and/or trans fats, which can increase the likelihood of developing type 2 diabetes and heart disease. Most baked goods and pastries are best avoided, unless you are a highly active child who can burn off those extra calories. The bottom line is that, for most of us, artificial sweeteners are a better choice than sugar, especially for people who have or are at risk for heart disease and diabetes.

Another source of extra sugar is energy bars. In general, I am not a big fan of these, other than for people who are engaged in strenuous exercise and need portable energy sources. Yes, energy bars may have healthy ingredients, such as whole grains or dried fruit. However, for most of us, better choices are the snacks that we show in our menus, with fruits and nuts or cheese, or yogurt and nuts. These choices will fill you up and keep you feeling satisfied longer, without the sugar spike from energy bars.

If you want to avoid the artificial sweeteners, fruit is a great source of natural sweetness and, of course, is a key part of the DASH plan. You can also try noncaloric natural sweeteners such as stevia. Many other natural sweeteners are based on fructose or sucrose, and thus have the same calories and contribution to blood sugar levels. Some examples are honey, agave, molasses, and maple syrup. With some of these foods, you can use a little less than with regular table sugar; however, it may not make a significant difference in calories. Again, with baked goods and pastries, less sugar means more starch, and therefore equal calories and blood glucose. Xylitol is a naturally occurring sugar alcohol that is becoming more common, and has similar benefits and concerns as other sugar alcohols.

Choosing the Best Carbs

Make a plan to choose great carbs. Think about which high-fiber foods you enjoy and take a list of them to the grocery store. Stock your pantry and fridge with all the options you love. If you want to avoid foods with artificial sweeteners, choose fruits for sweetness. It may take some planning, but once you get into your new habits, you won't even think about the higher-sugar options.

CHAPTER 9

The Skinny on Fats

What are the popular fats today? We hear a lot about omega-3s and monounsaturated fats. Everyone knows that we want to choose meats that are "lean" (if we eat meat). But it can be confusing to know what to eat, since "expert" nutrition recommendations have swung back and forth from saying limit your fat intake significantly to stating that fat isn't a villain; avoid all animal fats, but fish oil is great; butter is bad, but then margarine is worse. And on and on. I will try to help you understand which fats are good for you, and which ones should be avoided, especially for someone who is at risk for diabetes and heart disease.

The Contrarian Viewpoint

Some very popular fats that you will not find here include flax-seed (and its oil) and coconut oil. While much has been written about the health benefits of these fats, I am not convinced. We will choose fats that have been consumed by large groups of people for long periods of time and have been demonstrated to be associated with lower risk for heart disease.

Regarding flaxseed, this is not a foodstuff that has been extensively consumed by humans. The primary fat in flaxseed is alpha-linoleic acid (ALA), which is an omega-3 fatty acid. Some particular omega-3s are considered to be very healthful, specifically EPA and DHA. Flaxseed oil has been promoted as a plant source of omega-3s, which can be converted in the body to DHA and EPA. However, most evidence indicates that humans convert very little of the ALA into DHA and EPA. So this becomes less of a benefit. ALA is an essential fatty acid, but one that is unlikely to be deficient in a diet with a variety of heart-healthy fats. One recent study sought to learn about longer-term effects of flaxseed consumption. They were concerned that there could be problems with the production of red blood cells and kidney function. In the 4-week study, there were no immediate health problems. Flaxseed consumption did not lower blood pressure, did not lower cholesterol, but did raise harmful triglycerides. Some studies are suggesting that increased intake of ALA can raise the risk of prostate cancer. Flax and flaxseed oil are very susceptible to oxidation. And oxidation can be one of the initiators of some kinds of cancer. Proponents will say that the lignans in flax are strong antioxidants and so will counteract the oxidation potential of flaxseed oil. However, I remain concerned, since the lignans and the fats get separated during digestion, and each goes its own way in the body. So that leaves the linoleic acid subject to oxidation. To get a better understanding of this process, think of fats or oils going rancid. Is that a process you want going on in your body? It is, in fact, oxidation that causes fats to go rancid, and the fats that we are avoiding are more susceptible than others.

Coconut oil is almost 100% saturated fat, and makes a good foundation for increasing blood cholesterol levels. That is probably not your goal. And it is absorbed better than regular fats, since its short-chain fatty acids do not need to be broken down to be absorbable. Also, it is probably not your goal to eat fats that are better absorbed into your body, which would increase your net calories. In places in the world with high consumption of coconut oil, people tend to struggle with increased risks of obesity, diabetes, and heart disease. My experience at the navy hospital, counseling patients from the Philippines and Southeast Asia, showed that these were common problems. Even thin women were more likely to develop diabetes during pregnancy, especially if they cooked much of their food with coconut oil. The current thinking is that diets high in saturated fats are associated with increased risk for diabetes, which may in part be due to increased inflammatory response to these fats. Palm oil is another tropical fat that is high in saturated fats. Many food manufacturers have eliminated trans fats by replacing shortening with palm oil. And while we do certainly want to reduce trans fats in our diets, we do not want to increase saturated fats at the same time. Replacing one bad fat with another is not going to make us healthier.

Following the DASH diet will help reduce our "accidental" exposure to these bad fats. How? For most of us, who struggle with reaching and maintaining a healthy weight, there is not a lot of room in the DASH diet for the extra calories from baked goods and pastries. In the DASH Diet Weight Loss

Essential fatty acids are those that we must obtain from our diet, since our body cannot create them from other fats. The essential fats are alpha-linolenic acid and alpha-linoleic acid.

Solution, dessert is more likely to be fruit and/or some kind of no-added-sugar dairy food.

The Mainstream Viewpoint on Fats

What are heart-healthy fats? Fats that are the most heart-healthy are the long-chain fatty acids DHA (docosapentaenoic acid) and EPA (eicosapentaenoic acid) found primarily in cold-water fish, and the long-chain monounsaturated fat (MUFA) oleic acid, which is especially prevalent in nuts and olives. In the 1960s and 1970s, it was thought that polyunsaturated fats were the healthiest. People were strongly encouraged to choose vegetable oils such as corn oil and soybean oil. These are also known as omega-6 fatty acids. Now it is generally believed that excess consumption of the PUFA omega-6s, especially in relation to omega-3 fats, can increase inflammation.

However, the fish oil PUFAs, DHA and EPA, are believed to reduce inflammation. Consumption of fish oil supplements has been associated with lower rates of heart disease mortality and all-cause mortality. For many people, fish oil supplements are also helpful for reducing triglycerides, which is an early warning sign of developing insulin resistance.

Olive oil and other oils rich in MUFAs also reduce the risk of inflammation, and are associated with lower rates of heart disease and some types of cancer. For example, women in Greece who consume the highest amounts of olive oil have the lowest rates of breast cancer. And olive oil is a hallmark of the Mediterranean diet, which is well known to reduce heart disease mortality. (Actually, the DASH diet can be considered to be an Americanized version of the Mediterranean diet.)

While low-fat diets were strongly recommended by most

health guidelines in the late 1980s and most of the 1990s, the unintended consequences were found to be not so helpful as a health-promoting strategy. Fats were replaced by starches, which can be very healthy when they come from whole grains, but not so helpful in excess or from refined grains. Excess starches also are not beneficial in the sedentary American life-style when most of us have inadequate daily activity to burn off the calories. Starches break down to glucose, which can require lots of insulin to process. If people are not doing enough physical activity to have trained muscles that are efficient at burning and storing the carbs as glycogen, the excess glucose will get stored as fat, and mostly around the belly region. Many adults (and teens) have trouble efficiently responding to insulin to clean the glucose out of the blood, which is known as insulin resistance (IR). During the early stages of IR, the body will ramp up production of insulin. In children, insulin is a growth hormone, but in adults it is a fat-storage hormone. So eating more starchy foods than we burn off each day leads to more fat buildup, especially belly fat. If you look around at your family, friends, and community, you probably see way too many people who are at risk for developing insulin resistance and prediabetes. Now you can understand why we are in the middle of an escalating epidemic of diabetes.

But back to the fats. Including a moderate amount of fat in one's diet is beneficial. Fats help provide satiety and help us to avoid overeating. Fat helps with the absorption of fat-soluble vitamins and other plant nutrients, including many of the antioxidants. Foods that are especially rich in these heart-healthy fats include nuts, seeds, olives, and many cold-water ocean fish. Grass-fed beef can be another source of healthy fats.

The Bottom Line on Fats

We have all heard about which fats are unhealthy and should be avoided. Saturated and trans fats are definitely bad choices, since they help our bodies make more cholesterol and can increase inflammation. Further, saturated and trans may raise our risk for developing type 2 diabetes. The surprising thing is that we actually may be seeing more saturated fats in our diets than a few years ago. Shortening (a big source of trans fats) has been replaced in many foods with palm oil or coconut oil. As I have said, both of these foods are rich in saturated fats. Even worse, coconut oil is especially easy to digest and absorb. (Right. Just what we want—to do a better job of absorbing fats, instead of eliminating them.) While some authors may claim that these fats are healthful, that is still up for debate. Independent of my own clinical experience, in much of the Pacific islands, where coconut oil is the dominant fat, there are very high rates of obesity and elevated risk of diabetes.

Polyunsaturated fats (PUFAs) have been strongly promoted for heart health since the early 1960s. Now the evidence suggests that high intake of PUFAs is associated with increased inflammation. The exceptions to this are the marine long-chain PUFAs, also known as omega-3 fatty acids, we mentioned earlier, DHA and EPA.

The fats that we want to include in our diets include MUFAs such as those found in olive oil, peanut oil, and other nuts and seeds. Especially good sources include cashews, almonds, walnuts, and avocados. We also want to include the fatty cold-water fish that are rich in DHA and EPA, which include salmon, tuna, sardines, and swordfish. Since with the DASH Diet Weight Loss Solution you are doing a lot of the food preparation, it becomes easy to choose the right fats. And since the diet plan has far fewer baked goods and pastries than the typical diet, it also will remove hidden trans and saturated fats from your diet.

Think about how you will incorporate the healthy fats in your diet. Which types of fish will you choose for your meals? If you don't like fish, perhaps you should ask your physician or dietitian about adding a fish oil supplement. These supplements are associated with slightly "thinner" blood (that is, it is less likely to clot) and improved triglyceride levels. A major research study in Italy showed reduced rates of cardiovascular deaths, which was expected and, surprisingly, lower rates of cancer deaths with fish oil. These are the only supplements that have ever been shown to reduce heart disease mortality.

Consider which foods that are rich in monounsaturated fats you will choose. If you eat nuts, which are your favorites? Which cooking oils will you buy? If you have these key foods on hand, you will find it easy to be incorporating the healthiest fats.

CHAPTER 10

Rock Star Foods

Minerals are believed to be key to the DASH diet. Hidden in the main DASH foods are a rich variety of minerals. Of key importance are potassium, magnesium, and calcium. Sodium (from salt) is another important mineral, but one that we would like to keep relatively low. The DASH Diet Weight Loss Solution is also rich in vitamins, antioxidants, and other plant nutrients. Before we go any further, it is important to remember that it is the DASH diet food pattern that is important, not the isolated individual vitamins, minerals, or antioxidants.

DASH Minerals

It is believed that one of the key reasons that the DASH diet helps to lower blood pressure is that it is rich in foods that are high in potassium, magnesium, and calcium. Now, you may wonder, why not just make a supplement containing these minerals? Well, the researchers already tried that. And unfortunately, it didn't work. Most trials of vitamin supplementation have also been disappointing, with some even showing increased numbers of tumors with antioxidant supplements. New long-term research studies (one a very large European nutrition study and another a large study of women in Iowa) have shown that regular use of over-the-counter vitamin and mineral supplements is associated with an increased, not a lower, risk of death.

There is something about the whole DASH diet food pattern that makes for the health benefits. A diet that is high in fruits and vegetables, along with whole grains, nuts, seeds, and beans, is going to be very high in fiber and rich in antioxidants and other nutrients. Although there may be many weird theories about what to include in a diet, plant-based foods are almost always at the core of any diet plan. Certainly they are key to a healthy diet. Add in low-fat and nonfat dairy, and lean meats, fish, and poultry, and you have more of the beneficial minerals, with a meal plan that is still low in any of the concerning animal food components, such as saturated fat. Including healthy fats in your diet improves the heart-protective benefits, and may also reduce inflammation. Most of the DASH diet foods do double or triple duty in making a healthy diet.

Tables listing some of the DASH foods that are rich in potassium, magnesium, and calcium appear later in this chapter. In the following sections, we discuss the health benefits of each of the key food groups.

Fruits and Vegetables

Fruits and vegetables, of course, are great sources of minerals, vitamins, and fiber. They are usually some of the most nutrient-packed foods, and many are very rich in minerals, especially potassium.

Whole Grains

While whole grains are not very high in minerals, they are good sources, and do contain small amounts of some of the minerals that are needed in trace amounts. They are one of the most important sources of magnesium in our diets. And of course, whole grains have many other benefits, including fiber and antioxidant vitamins, and they are important sources of B vitamins.

Nuts, Beans, and Seeds

Way back in the 1990s, when fat was "bad," we threw the baby out with the bathwater. Not all fats are problematic, and nuts and seeds are certainly wonderful sources of all kinds of nutrients, including heart-healthy fats. Add in the protein in nuts, and you also have a powerful tool to quench hunger. Nuts and seeds are very good sources of key DASH minerals, especially potassium and magnesium.

Beans, of course, are rich in fiber and protein, and they are also good sources of important vitamins and minerals. Beans are wonderful sources of both potassium and magnesium, which are key to the blood pressure–lowering benefits of the DASH diet. Since beans are often used as meat alternatives, it is fortuitous that they are also rich in iron.

Low-Fat and Nonfat Dairy

Dairy is one of the key DASH diet foods. When the first study was done, one of the three test groups had a diet with extra amounts of fruits and vegetables, without adding in extra dairy. They did not see the blood pressure–lowering effect of the full DASH plan. Of course, we all know that dairy is the most important source of calcium in the typical American diet. But did you also know that dairy foods are also very rich in potassium and magnesium? Yes, milk has about 125 milligrams of sodium as well, but we don't want to exclude it from our diets in the pursuit of "low salt."

If you are sensitive to lactose or milk proteins, you can choose dairy substitutes. Take care to choose products with equal calcium and vitamin D to their real dairy counterparts. (For more information on food intolerances and allergies, see Appendix A.)

Lean Meats, Fish, and Poultry

When it comes to minerals, the protein-rich foods are important "Rock Stars." Beef is our best source for iron since it is much better absorbed from meat than from plant foods, about 28% versus only 4%. Beef and many types of fish are great sources of potassium. Additionally, meat, fish, and poultry have many other very important trace minerals that boost our health. Add all of these healthy nutrients to the benefits of building and maintaining muscle, providing satiety to meals, and we can see that they can be part of a healthy diet. Certainly we are not insisting that animal foods have to be part of a healthy plan, but providing flexibility for those who do enjoy them. One of the main concepts behind the DASH diet was to take the benefits of a vegetarian diet and make the plan flexible enough to appeal to most of us. So no proselytizing on this side, choose more plant-based foods and enjoy!

Mining for Your Best Mineral Sources

Below are lists of key foods that are rich in potassium, magnesium, and calcium. While these tables are not comprehensive, they will help give you an idea of important foods to incorporate into your diet for better health and weight loss. You should note that we did not include oxalate-rich foods such as spinach, Swiss chard, and beet greens, even though they do contain calcium, because of the very poor absorption of the minerals in those foods. It doesn't mean that these are bad foods; it just means that they aren't going contribute to your calcium needs.

Calcium-Rich Foods

Dairy: milk, yogurt, cottage cheese, cheese

Vegetables: broccoli, kale, bok choi

Beans: soybeans, tofu

Seafood: sardines and other fish with bones

Potassium-Rich Foods

Vegetables: asparagus, artichoke, avocado, bamboo shoot, beans, beet, broccoli, Brussels sprouts, carrot, cauliflower, celery, kale, mushroom, okra, potato, pumpkin, seaweed, spinach, squash (winter), sweet potato, tomato, turnip greens

Fruits: apple, apricot, avocado, banana, cantaloupe, date, dried fruit, grapefruit, honeydew, kiwifruit, orange, peach, pear, prune, strawberry, tangerine

Nuts: almonds, Brazil nuts, cashews, chestnuts, filberts, hazelnuts, peanuts, pecans, pumpkin seeds, sunflower seeds, walnuts

Cereals and breads: bran cereals, Mueslix, pumpernickel bread

Meat and poultry: pork and, at lower amounts, beef, poultry

Seafood: halibut, salmon, cod, clams, tuna, rockfish, rainbow trout, lobster, crab

Dairy: milk, yogurt

Miscellaneous: coffee, molasses, tea, tofu

Magnesium-Rich Foods

Fruits and vegetables: avocado, banana, beans, beet greens, black-eyed peas, cassava, fig, lentils, okra, potato with skin, raisins, seaweed, spinach, Swiss chard, wax beans

Whole grains: amaranth, barley, bran, brown rice, buckwheat, bulgur, granola, millet, oats, rye, triticale, whole wheat, wild rice

Dairy: milk, yogurt

Nuts: almonds, Brazil nuts, cashews, flaxseeds, hazel nuts, macadamia nuts, peanuts, pecans, pistachios, pumpkin seeds, sesame seeds, soybeans, sunflower seeds, walnuts

Seafood: salmon, tuna, lobster, halibut, cod

Drinking to Your Health

In addition to all these nutrients, of course, we all need to get sufficient fluid every day. There are many ways to accomplish this, and most are absolutely great with the DASH diet. And everyone wants to know what to drink when following this plan. The good news is that you have lots of options. My best advice is to drink when you are thirsty. Avoid sugar-laden beverages. The following are some myths that may surprise you.

Fluid Myths

1. We all need at least 8 glasses of water each day.

   False. Depending on how much we sweat, most of us need 6–8 (8-ounce) glasses of fluid each day. This includes the water that comes from food, such as fruits and vegetables.

2. Caffeinated beverages don't count as water since they are dehydrating.

False. You will excrete a tiny amount of extra water with caffeinated beverages, but they still contribute to your total daily intake of water.

3. Drink water with your meals to feel fuller.

False. Research shows that drinking water with meals does almost nothing to quench hunger. However, eating foods that are high in water content, including (low-sodium) soups, fruits, and vegetables, does help you avoid overeating.

Beverages	Recommended?	Suggestions
Coffee	Yes	Add skim milk. Make it a latte and it becomes another dairy serving. Use only noncaloric sweeteners.
Tea	Yes	Add skim milk. Use only noncaloric sweeteners.
Soda, with sugar	No	
Soda, sugar-free	Yes	
Packaged powder beverages	Yes, artificially sweetened only	
Milk	Skim, or nonfat	Make hot chocolate with skim milk, cocoa powder, and noncaloric sweetener.
Wine	Yes, but not in the first 14 days	Red wine is best. Limit to 3½ ounces for women, double that for men. Each glass replaces one fruit serving.

(Continued)

Beverages	Recommended?	Suggestions
Beer	Okay, but not in the first 14 days	Each regular beer replaces 2 grain servings. A light beer replaces 1 grain.
Other alcoholic beverages	Okay, but not in the first 14 days	1 shot replaces one grain.
Smoothies	Occasionally okay, but not in the first 14 days	Count as your dairy and fruit servings.*
Water	Yes	In some areas, it can be a significant source of calcium.

* In general, choose whole fruits and vegetables to get the bulk, and slow digestion. Fruit that has been pulverized in smoothies will contribute to a "sugar rush," which is something most of us want to avoid. (In a blender, the fruit fiber is pulverized, significantly reducing its effectiveness, and the sugar is released from the fruit cells, making it much easier to absorb quickly. A little of this happens during chewing, but not at all to the extent that it does when fruit is blended.) Limit smoothies to special occasions or avoid altogether.

PART III

The Healthiest Diet, How It Keeps *You* Healthier

CHAPTER 11

Taking It to Heart, with the DASH Diet

Heart disease is the number one killer of women and men, with stroke being the third. In 2010, cardiovascular disease (CVD) cost the United States about $444 billion. About 83 million adult Americans (33%) have some kind of heart disease. Each year, about 735,000 people have heart attacks. Another 795,000 have strokes. There are 68 million who have high blood pressure (hypertension), while another 25% of adults have prehypertension.

Heart disease clearly is a significant problem for large numbers of Americans. Some people may think that they have a strong family history of early heart disease so there is not much they can do about it. Others think that if it is inevitable, they would rather not make any changes in their lifestyle that might diminish their quality of life. However, very few people would like to suffer the lingering effects of a debilitating stroke or live with heart failure. Unfortunately, we don't get a choice about how our own personal heart disease might play out. So perhaps we should do something now to have better heart health.

The most obvious risks for heart disease include high blood pressure and high cholesterol. Of course, there are additional risks, which we can divide into those that you can and those that you cannot control.

Heart Disease Risks

Not Under Your Control	Under Your Control
Family history of early heart disease	Hypertension
Age 45+ for men and 55+ for women	High cholesterol and triglycerides
	Low HDL
	Obesity
	Smoking
	Diabetes
	Sedentary lifestyle

Since most of the aspects of heart disease risk are under our control, we may as well do something about them. We all want to stay healthy as we get older and to live long, active lives. If you have a family history of early heart disease, then you are probably also at elevated risk. You will want to pay special attention to the risks that you can control. It can be easy to blame heredity for health issues, but just because nature gave you a loaded gun, it doesn't mean you have to pull the trigger by having a poor lifestyle. For most of us, our choices will impact whether we have heart disease and how early it will strike.

If we have high blood pressure, high cholesterol, high tri-glycerides, low HDL, and/or diabetes, we need to be complying with our doctor's recommendations for medication and lifestyle changes. If we are overweight or obese, we can take actions to work on losing weight. We can give up smoking and become more physically active.

Of course, one of the most important things that we can do is to follow the DASH diet. DASH was originally developed specifically to lower blood pressure without medication. The research studies were entitled "Dietary Approaches to Stop Hypertension." And that it does. It also helps people respond better to their blood pressure medication, if they aren't able to eliminate it entirely. Many people have told us that their doctors were unable to get their blood pressure under control until they started the DASH diet.

Fortunately, the DASH diet also lowers total cholesterol. Evidence shows that lower-carb diets will help raise the good cholesterol, while helping to lower triglycerides. The DASH diet has also been shown to help reduce the risk of developing type 2 diabetes. Cutting out the junk carbs of highly processed starchy foods, along with including all of the core DASH foods, will slow the progression of the disease for many people, and will please most endo-crinologists. After all, type 2 diabetes is a consequence of not responding well to insu-lin, which eventually exhausts the body's ability to produce enough insulin. Consuming less starch, as you do with the DASH Diet Weight Loss

Food Sources of Bad or Good Cholesterol?

I am often asked which foods have bad cholesterol, so that it can be avoided. Foods contain plain cholesterol. The good and bad refer to how the cholesterol is packaged in our blood.

Solution, will help avoid overtaxing the body's insulin-producing cells. Losing weight helps many people respond better to insulin, further helping to stave off diabetes or making it easier to control.

Smoking cessation is a challenge for many people. While changes in public policy have made it more difficult to smoke in public and have significantly raised the cost of smoking, about 20% of the adult U.S. population still smoke. It is more prevalent in younger adults than older ones. Even in young people, smoking just one cigarette can increase artery stiffness by 25% with physical activity. This can lead to higher blood pressure and arteries that are more prone to clog with cholesterol. Additionally, the blood of smokers carries less oxygen, is more prone to clot, and forces the heart to work harder. The risk of an ischemic stroke (one where a clot prevents blood flow to part of the brain, resulting in death of brain cells) is almost doubled in smokers.

Fortunately, the benefits of smoking cessation occur very quickly. Within 12 hours, your blood pressure and pulse rate will return to normal, as will your blood oxygen levels. Within 2 days, your senses of taste and smell start returning. After 1 year, your risk of having a heart attack or stroke has been cut in half compared to smokers. Within 5 years, the risk of a fatal heart attack has decreased 61%, while the risk of a fatal stroke is reduced 42%. After about 15 years, your risk of heart attack and stroke is the same as for someone who has never smoked.

Losing weight, if you are overweight or obese, will help to reduce your risk of heart disease. Being overweight means that you are more likely to have high cholesterol, high triglycerides, and low HDL. You are more likely to have high blood pressure and to respond less well to insulin. Independent of these risks, even small increases in weight can significantly raise your risk of having a heart attack. Middle-aged women who have BMIs between 23 and 25 (which is still in the healthy range) are 50% more likely to have coronary heart disease, while men whose BMI is 25 to 29 (overweight status) have a 72% increased risk.

Heart Health Targets

Many people know their heart health numbers. Do you? Let's review them here.

Blood Pressure

	Systolic Blood Pressure	Diastolic Blood Pressure
Healthy blood pressure	Less than 120 and greater than 90	Less than 80 and higher than 60
Prehypertension	120 to 139	80 to 89
Hypertension, stage 1	140 to 159	90 to 99
Hypertension, stage 2	160 or higher	100 or higher

The top number in blood pressure is the systolic blood pressure (SBP) and is the pressure when your heart beats (pumps); the bottom number is the diastolic blood pressure (DBP) and is the pressure when your heart rests between beats. Healthy blood pressure is related to having relatively elastic blood vessels that are able to flex when the heart beats. Stiffer vessels are associated with increased blood pressure. Less flexible arteries can continue to worsen, leading to hardening of the arteries. Stiffer arteries and veins are more likely to become clogged with cholesterol buildup, which can impair blood flow to all parts of the body, including the kidneys, brain, arms, and legs.

High blood pressure can lead to kidney failure, heart failure, strokes, aneurysms, angina, reduced cognitive function, eye damage, impotence, and peripheral vascular disease.

Unfortunately, only half of the people with high blood pressure have it under control. Causes of poor control include not having been diagnosed, failure to take prescribed medication, and noncompliance with recommended lifestyle changes. The diet and exercise guidance in this book will support improving your blood pressure.

Lipids

Lipids is the scientific name for fats, and in this case we are referring specifically to the fats in your blood. The two most important types of fat include cholesterol and triglycerides. Cholesterol is further broken down into low-density cholesterol (LDL), high-density cholesterol (HDL), and very-low-density cholesterol (VLDL), which is not commonly reported on your lab reports. LDL is considered the "bad" cholesterol, since it tends to deposit cholesterol along the linings of your blood vessels. HDL is the "good" cholesterol, because it cleans up the deposits. Having high HDL means that these particles are carrying lots of cholesterol away from your arteries, and sending it to the liver for removal.

Classifications of Blood Lipid Levels

Total Cholesterol

Desirable: <200

Borderline high: 200–239

High: 240+

LDL Cholesterol

Desirable with CVD: <70

Optimal: <100

Near or above optimal: 100–129

Borderline high: 130–159

High: 160–189

Very high: 190+

HDL Cholesterol

Low: <40

High (desirable): 60+

Triglycerides (Triacylglyerols)

Normal: <150

Borderline high: 150–199

High: 200–499

Very high: 500+

Triglycerides are other types of fats that are concerning for heart health. They tend to deposit in veins and arteries, similar to LDL. Further, elevated triglycerides can be an early warning sign that you are at higher risk for developing type 2 diabetes. When your blood sugar stays higher than normal for an extended time, the liver will pick up some of the excess sugar. After the liver has enough sugar stored as glycogen, it will then start converting the excess sugar into fatty acids, which are combined into triglycerides, much of which are packaged and pumped back out into the bloodstream. Unfortunately, these packaged triglycerides soak up cholesterol from the HDL, reducing its ability to send the cholesterol back to the liver for elimination. Thus, triglycerides are both a symptom of developing insulin resistance and a problem for heart health.

Your physician may have different goals for you than the general population guidelines. However, these are the standard goals for blood lipids. People with higher risks for heart disease may be asked to reduce their LDL lower than the standard guidelines. Having diabetes is one of the factors that increase your risk for heart disease, so there are stricter guidelines for people with diabetes.

Having elevated levels of blood lipids goes hand in hand with high blood pressure to damage arteries and veins, and increases the risk for all of the same diseases as hypertension. It is important for us to emphasize the higher risk for heart attack, fatal or not, associated with high cholesterol.

Fortunately, the DASH diet supports improving cholesterol levels through lower intake of saturated fats, increased intake of calcium, and higher intake of fiber. The body uses saturated fats and trans fats to make cholesterol. Fiber and calcium can help reduce the amount of fat that your body absorbs. Choosing lean meats, limiting dairy fat, and avoiding plant sources of saturated fats (such as palm oil and coconut oil) are all key DASH strategies for lower cholesterol. We worry more about the intake of these unhealthy fats than we do about dietary cholesterol, since we consume about 100 times more saturated fat than we do cholesterol. Additionally, the reduced starch intake from the DASH Diet Weight Loss Solution will help lower triglycerides and reduce the amount of cholesterol that your body makes. Who knew? A high-carb diet fires up production of the enzyme (HMG CoA reductase) that helps in the production of cholesterol in your liver. A higher-carb diet depresses the level of good cholesterol and raises the level of bad cholesterol. None of these are desired, so cutting back on those starchy foods will have many benefits for heart health.

Reducing Your Personal Risk for Heart Disease

Most of the heart disease risks are under your control. Family history, sex, and age are not. So focus on the things that you can change, most of which are addressed with the DASH Diet Weight Loss Solution. Follow this plan and work in concert with your physician to control your blood pressure, cholesterol and triglycerides, and blood sugar. Reach and maintain a healthy weight. Become more physically active and quit smoking.

CHAPTER 12

DASHing Your Risk of Diabetes

There are three blood sugar diseases that go together: insulin resistance, metabolic syndrome, and type 2 diabetes. Insulin resistance sounds like "medical talk," which it is, but it is very important to understand the process that can lead to developing type 2 diabetes. About 25 million Americans have the disease. Another 35% of adult Americans have prediabetes. That figure jumps to 50% of people who are 65 or older. In the United States in 2007, diabetes was estimated to have cost $175 billion. It is associated with increased risk of kidney failure, blindness, heart disease, and amputations.

On a more practical level, most of us are fearful of developing diabetes. While it is becoming more common and treatable, and almost all of us know someone dear to us who has diabetes, we still don't want to have it controlling our lives. If you have a strong family history of diabetes, or if you have some of the early warning signs, such as high triglycerides, expanding waistline, or a diagnosis of prediabetes, then you will appreciate having a plan to do something about it.

Genetics or heredity can play a strong factor in whether you are likely to develop diabetes. Beyond a family history of diabetes, several racial and ethnic groups are at higher risk for developing type 2 diabetes, including Latinos and Hispanics, Native Americans and Alaskan Natives, African-Americans, South Asians, and Pacific Islanders. Fortunately, research has shown that improving eating habits and exercising moderately can reverse or prevent the onset of diabetes. Knowing that you are at risk can help motivate you to move more and eat better.

How Are Type 1 and Type 2 Diabetes Different?

With type 1 diabetes, the body quickly and completely loses the ability to produce insulin. Typically, this happens in childhood, but it can strike at any age. It is also known as juvenile diabetes or insulin-dependent diabetes. People with type 1 diabetes have to use insulin with every meal. It is also possible for people with type 1 diabetes to develop insulin resistance later in life.

With type 2 diabetes, the body slowly stops being able to produce enough insulin. Insulin resistance is a hallmark. Most often it develops later in life. It is also known as adult-onset diabetes and non-insulin-dependent diabetes (even though some people with type 2 will need insulin).

Insulin is the body's hormone that helps to move blood sugar into the cells, particularly into muscles. When you have a meal with sugar or starch, your blood glucose (blood sugar) rises and triggers the pancreas to produce insulin. Insulin resistance is the condition in which your body stops responding to insulin as efficiently as it did when you were younger (although, unfortunately, this condition can occur in children and teens). When your body doesn't respond as well to the insulin, your pancreas pumps out higher levels to try to keep blood sugar under control. Over time, this overproduction can wear out the cells that produce insulin, and then you won't be able to produce enough to keep blood sugar under control.

The liver normally contains some sugar stored as glycogen, but it can hold only a limited amount. If blood sugar is still high, the liver will convert the excess into triglycerides (see Chapter 11). Some of these triglycerides are stored in the liver, which can cause fatty liver disease. And some get packaged into particles and sent back into the bloodstream, where they can soak up cholesterol from the HDL (good cholesterol), reducing its ability to send the cholesterol to the liver for elimination.

Some of the first symptoms that will be noticed by your doctor might be slightly high glucose and/or high triglycerides. You might have noticed that you have gained extra weight around the middle. Sorry, but yes, that is an important sign that you are at risk for developing diabetes. Sadly, the one area where your body still responds well to insulin is in the fat cells around your belly region. Excess sugar gets soaked up by these fat cells, and gets converted into more fat.

Some of the lifestyle factors that can provoke insulin resistance are physical inactivity and long-term consumption of excess calories, especially from sugar and starch, both of which would, of course, be related to overweight and obesity. The good news is that research has shown that getting on track with healthy eating, losing as little as 7% of body weight, and adding moderate activity (30 minutes five times per week) can reverse or prevent insulin resistance.

Definitions of Diabetes and Insulin Resistance

Normal blood sugar is less than 100 when fasting, and optimal healthy blood sugar is about 75 to 80. Prediabetes is when the blood sugar is between 100 and 125 when fasting. This can also be called insulin resistance, impaired glucose tolerance, or impaired fasting glucose, depending on which test was used to diagnose it. People are diagnosed with diabetes if their fasting blood sugar has been 126 or higher on one or more occasions, or if their nonfasting blood sugar is over 200. Another measure is A1c (which is glycosylated hemoglobin), which if over 6.5 is considered to be indicative of diabetes. A1c measures the level of sugar attached to your blood hemoglobin, which is related to how high your blood sugar has been over the past three months.

Metabolic Syndrome

Metabolic syndrome is related to insulin resistance. It is also called Syndrome X, insulin resistance syndrome, or dysmetabolic syndrome. The cluster of symptoms, including elevated blood pressure, elevated blood sugar, high triglycerides, low HDL, and high waist circumference, are related to how your body processes blood sugar. Fortunately, the lifestyle changes to manage this syndrome are exactly the same as for improving insulin sensitivity, lowering blood pressure, and improving blood lipids. Controlling all these issues reduces your risk of heart disease and diabetes. The DASH Diet Weight Loss Solution, with lower levels of starchy foods and plenty of exercise, will help improve the symptoms and interrelated physical problems at their most fundamental level.

Metabolic Syndrome Diagnosis (U.S.)
Includes 3 or More of the Following

Triglycerides	Over 150
Waist circumference	Over 40 inches (102 cm) for men Over 35 inches (88 cm) for women
Low HDL	Less than 40 mg/dL for men Less than 50 mg/dL for women
Elevated blood pressure	Greater than 130 SBP or 85 DBP or on medication for blood pressure
Elevated blood glucose	Fasting glucose greater than 110 mg/dL

CHAPTER 13

The DASH Diet for the Science Geeks

While the DASH Diet Weight Loss Solution is relatively intuitive to follow, many people still want to get into the details of why and how it works.

The original premise of the DASH diet was to lower blood pressure. The research study was called Dietary Approaches to Stop Hypertension. One of the guiding principles was that vegetarian diets were known to be associated with lower blood pressure. The researchers wanted to take the best elements of vegetarian diets and develop a dietary pattern that would be flexible enough to accommodate the food preferences of most Americans, while still being a very healthy diet.

Eating patterns that were rich in potassium, magnesium, and calcium were known to be associated with lower blood pressure. It would seem to be an easy solution to just add dietary supplements containing these minerals in order to promote healthier blood pressure. In fact, many studies had been done looking at the effect of dietary supplements with these minerals. Unfortunately, these studies did not show a consistent benefit from pills.

When you look at dietary patterns that are abundant in potassium, calcium, and magnesium, they also tend to be rich in vitamins C and D and high in fiber. The researchers decided to develop a program based on food patterns, rather than dietary components.

When the first DASH diet studies were being developed in the early 1990s, the conventional nutrition wisdom held that diets rich in starches, especially from grains, and lower in fats and proteins were the key to health and reduced obesity. Of course, we now know that didn't work out so well. But this philosophy shaped the original design of the DASH diet.

For the initial studies, the targets for caloric contributions for the DASH diet were 55% carbohydrate, 18% protein, and 27% fat. The salt content at 3,000 milligrams per day was much higher than would be used today, since there was no RDA for sodium at that time—there was just a recommendation for a minimum amount that was deemed to be adequate and safe. Further, the researchers wanted to evaluate the effect of the dietary pattern, not sodium reduction, on blood pressure.

The key daily nutrient targets were to have at least 4,700 milligrams of potassium, 1,250 milligrams of calcium, 500 milligrams of magnesium, and 31 grams of fiber. In practice, the research diet was only able to reach 4,500 milligrams of potassium. The targets for calcium and magnesium were much easier to reach, and the target for fiber was exceeded.

Another concern of the researchers was that certain ethnic groups had higher rates of hypertension, and were more likely to have serious health complications from elevated blood pressure.[1] So when choosing study subjects, they included African-

Americans at numbers higher than their representation in the general population. And certain regions of the country are more likely to be affected by consequences of hypertension. A region of the country, mostly in the Southeast, following the lower Appalachian Mountains over toward Texas, is called the Stroke Belt.[2] Fortunately, two of the sites chosen for the study were in the Stroke Belt, at Duke University in North Carolina and the Pennington Biomedical Research Center in Louisiana. Thus, the DASH diet was tested with the aim of targeting the groups that were especially hard hit with high blood pressure. If it could work for the most vulnerable people, then the DASH diet would certainly be a valuable diet plan.

Not so surprisingly, since we now know that DASH has been rated as the best and the healthiest diet plan, it did work to lower blood pressure, even in the people with the highest likelihood of having high blood pressure. In the initial study, there were three arms. The first group ate a typical American diet, the second group consumed the typical diet with additional fruits and vegetables, and the third group followed the DASH plan, which contained the extra fruits and vegetables and extra low-fat dairy foods.

Because the purpose of the study was to evaluate the effect of the food pattern on blood pressure, the participants were not allowed to lose (or gain) weight during the study. Weight change would have muddied the waters when it came to evaluating the effect of the diet plan on hypertension. Losing weight, on its own, can improve blood pressure.

Interestingly, the group with just added fruits and vegetables did not have an improvement in blood pressure. It was only the group following the entire DASH diet plan, including the additional dairy, which showed an improvement in blood pressure. Many times the DASH diet is oversimplified and merely described as a plan rich in fruits and veggies. However, this misses the key balance of the overall plan. Without the calcium and vitamin D from dairy, the plan did not work. On the other hand, many people think that DASH is just another low-sodium plan. However, in this first study, sodium was significantly higher than the current DRI recommendations.

And yet significant reductions in blood pressure were seen in study participants who had hypertension. SBP was reduced by 11.4 mm Hg and DBP by 5.5 mm Hg.[3] Without lowering sodium. Without losing weight. The DASH diet, complete with dairy and extra fruits and vegetables, was able to improve blood pressure, even without other important lifestyle changes.

A later study was designed to evaluate the benefit of sodium reduction in addition to the DASH food pattern. It was entitled the DASH-sodium study.[4] This study showed that further reductions in sodium could be helpful for improving blood pressure for many people with high blood pressure, especially African-American women and older people in general.[5] Since the DASH diet already lowers blood pressure without sodium restriction, the benefit of lowering salt intake was much stronger in people who were eating a typical American diet. The DASH diet with 3,500 milligrams of sodium provided about the same degree of blood pressure reduction as the typical diet with sodium reduced to 1,500 milligrams. The DASH diet thus provides some protection for occasionally having higher-salt meals.

DASH has been shown to lower total cholesterol and LDL cholesterol.[6] There was a slight reduction in HDL cholesterol and no change in triglycerides. However, it should be remembered that the earliest DASH studies were relatively high in starchy foods, which are associated with depressing HDL levels and contributing to triglyceride levels.

A study of the DASH diet with patients who had metabolic

syndrome (insulin resistance, low HDL, elevated blood pressure, and/or high triglycerides) showed improvements in LDL, HDL, triglycerides, fasting blood glucose, and blood pressure.[7]

Because the original DASH diet was developed at the time when high-starch, low-fat diets were thought to be beneficial, starch is at the core of the original DASH research. As more research in the 2000s was showing that there might be benefit to lowering the starch content of the diet, the DASH researchers decided to evaluate this modification.[8] They evaluated replacing starch with either protein-rich foods or fats rich in mono-unsaturated fats (MUFAs). This study was done under the name "OMNI-Heart (Optimal Macro-Nutrient Intake Heart) Trial."[9] The results showed that both substitutions (protein and MUFAs) were better than the original DASH food pattern for lowering blood pressure (especially in people with hypertension) and in lowering triglycerides. The people who were on the plan with the higher level of protein reported that their hunger levels were lower than those on either the higher-fat plan or the starch-rich plan. This could not be explained by differences in appetite hormone levels.[10]

Studies of Lower-Carb Diets and Weight Loss

I will briefly discuss a few of the studies that were run with the purpose of showing the negative effects of the high-protein, low-carb diets. One of the first studies was sponsored in part by the American Heart Association, looking to discourage people from following the Atkins diet. This study, under the direction of Bonnie Brehm, PhD, RD, provided guidance to about half of the participants on how to follow an Atkins-style diet while the other participants were provided advice on following a reduced-calorie, relatively low-fat diet.[11] The participants on the very low-carb diet plan lost more weight and more fat weight. Both groups had similar improvements in markers of heart health. Another similar study also found improved weight loss with the low-carb plan, as measured at 3 and 6 months, but with comparable results by one year, as compared with a conventional low-fat diet plan.[12] Most markers of heart health and glucose control were improved similarly in both groups. However, in the low-carb group, HDL and triglycerides were significantly improved.

Don Layman, PhD, professor emeritus from the University of Illinois, has focused much of his research on helping to understand the effectiveness of higher-protein and lower-carbohydrate diets. His research has shown that they are beneficial in terms of promoting improved weight loss, while being heart healthy, and improving lean body mass, which is associated with faster metabolism.[13] Dr. Layman has shown that having a higher protein intake, around 125 grams per day, will help with improving body composition (reduced fat loss versus muscle mass loss) while dieting, or help to preserve muscle mass for those dieting plus adding moderate exercise.[14]

For people who carry their excess weight around their middle and/or have some degree of insulin resistance, carbohydrate restriction is recommended by many endocrinologists.[15] It appears to be beneficial even independent of weight loss. This is a major contrast with the dietary advice in the 1990s, when the typical recommendations for people with type 2 diabetes included 55% of the calories coming from carbs.

Additional Health Benefits from the DASH Diet

Because the DASH diet has been found to be so healthful, many researchers have been interested in knowing what the long-term benefits would be of following the diet. There are several ongoing studies that have been following people for long periods of time and have been tracking their food intake and health history. Many of the reports on the long-term benefits of DASH come from these studies, especially the Nurses' Health Study (NHS) and the Male Health Professionals Study (MHPS), which have been following their participants for over 20 years.

From these studies, we have learned that people who follow the DASH diet for much of their life have lower rates of strokes, heart attacks, and heart failure. An evaluation of the NHS showed that women who followed an eating pattern conforming to the DASH diet, over 24 years of monitoring, had significantly lower rates of heart disease and stroke.[16] A study following 39,000 men aged 45–79 years old, for 7 years, found a 22% lower risk of developing heart failure if they ate a diet that was consistent with the DASH eating plan.[17] A separate study, following the health history of 36,000 women over 7 years, showed that women who followed an eating pattern consistent with the DASH diet were 37% less likely to develop heart failure.[18]

Following over 40,000 men for over 20 years, in the Health Professionals Follow-Up Study, it was seen that men who followed an eating pattern that conformed to the DASH diet were less likely to develop type 2 diabetes.[19] Men who were heavier were more likely to see the benefits in risk reduction. A similar study of 37,000 women evaluated the effect of healthy diets rich in fruits and vegetables and saw reduced risk of type 2 diabetes in women.[20]

The DASH diet has also been shown to help preserve kidney function in women with early signs of impaired function.[21] Further, the risk of developing kidney stones was about

55% reduced in men and women following a DASH eating pattern.[22] This study was especially powerful since it followed about 46,000 men for 18 years, and 196,000 women for 14 to 18 years. This reduction in risk came in spite of the fact that the people following the DASH eating pattern had much higher intake of calcium and oxalic acid, which historically were discouraged for people with a history of kidney stones.

From the NHS we have learned that women who follow a DASH-style eating pattern are less likely to develop estrogen receptor negative (ER-) breast cancer.[23] Following a lower-carb diet also reduces the risk. Colorectal cancer rates have been shown to be about 20% lower in people following the DASH plan.[24]

Food patterns that are rich in plant-based foods are well known to be very good sources of antioxidants. And a study performed by a group outside of the original DASH consortium found that the DASH diet was very effective at lowering the oxidative stress of obesity, which may be a factor in improving blood pressure.[25] A report by the DASH group found that they were able to show reduced markers of oxidative stress and increased antibodies for oxidized LDL cholesterol in one of their studies.[26] The DASH diet also appears to improve bone health, and has been shown to be associated with lower markers of bone turnover, which is associated with osteoporosis.[27]

Notes

1. Rationale and design of the Dietary Approaches to Stop Hypertension (DASH) trial. A multicenter controlled-feeding study of dietary patterns to lower blood pressure. Sacks FM, Obarzanek E, Windhauser MM, Svetkey LP, Vollmer WM, McCullough M, Karanja N, Lin PH, Steele P, Proschan MA, et al. *Annals of Epidemiology.* 1995 Mar;5(2):108–18.

2. The complete list of states in the Stroke Belt is Alabama, Arkansas, Georgia, Indiana, Kentucky, Louisiana, Mississippi, North Carolina,

South Carolina, Tennessee, and Virginia. http://www.nhlbi.nih.gov/health/prof/heart/other/sb_spec.pdf. Accessed on February 6, 2012.

3. A clinical trial of the effects of dietary patterns on blood pressure. DASH Collaborative Research Group. Appel LJ, Moore TJ, Obarzanek E, Vollmer WM, Svetkey LP, Sacks FM, Bray GA, Vogt TM, Cutler JA, Windhauser MM, Lin PH, Karanja N. *New England Journal of Medicine.* 1997 Apr 17;336(16):1117–24.

4. Effects on blood pressure of reduced dietary sodium and the Dietary Approaches to Stop Hypertension (DASH) diet. DASH-Sodium Collaborative Research Group. Sacks FM, Svetkey LP, Vollmer WM, Appel LJ, Bray GA, Harsha D, Obarzanek E, Conlin PR, Miller ER 3rd, Simons-Morton DG, Karanja N, Lin PH. *New England Journal of Medicine.* 2001 Jan 4;344(1):3–10.

5. Effects of diet and sodium intake on blood pressure: subgroup analysis of the DASH-sodium trial. Vollmer WM, Sacks FM, Ard J, Appel LJ, Bray GA, Simons-Morton DG, Conlin PR, Svetkey LP, Erlinger TP, Moore TJ, Karanja N; DASH-Sodium Trial Collaborative Research Group. *Annals of Internal Medicine.* 2001 Dec 18;135(12):1019–28.

6. Effects on blood lipids of a blood pressure–lowering diet: the Dietary Approaches to Stop Hypertension (DASH) Trial. Obarzanek E, Sacks FM, Vollmer WM, Bray GA, Miller ER 3rd, Lin PH, Karanja NM, Most-Windhauser MM, Moore TJ, Swain JF, Bales CW, Proschan MA; DASH Research Group. *American Journal of Clinical Nutrition.* 2001 Jul;74(1):80–89.

7. Beneficial effects of a Dietary Approaches to Stop Hypertension eating plan on features of the metabolic syndrome. Azadbakht L, Mirmiran P, Esmaillzadeh A, Azizi T, Azizi F. *Diabetes Care.* 2005 Dec;28(12):2823–31.

8. Rationale and design of the Optimal Macro-Nutrient Intake Heart Trial to Prevent Heart Disease (OMNI-Heart). Carey VJ, Bishop L, Charleston J, Conlin P, Erlinger T, Laranjo N, McCarron P, Miller E, Rosner B, Swain J, Sacks FM, Appel LJ. *Clinical Trials.* 2005;2(6):529–37.

9. Effects of protein, monounsaturated fat, and carbohydrate intake on blood pressure and serum lipids: results of the OmniHeart randomized trial. Appel LJ, Sacks FM, Carey VJ, Obarzanek E, Swain JF, Miller ER 3rd, Conlin PR, Erlinger TP, Rosner BA, Laranjo NM, Charleston J, McCarron P, Bishop LM; OmniHeart Collaborative

Research Group. *Journal of the American Medical Association.* 2005 Nov 16;294(19):2455–64.

10. Associations between macronutrient intake and self-reported appetite and fasting levels of appetite hormones: results from the Optimal Macronutrient Intake Trial to Prevent Heart Disease. Beasley JM, Ange BA, Anderson CA, Miller ER 3rd, Erlinger TP, Holbrook JT, Sacks FM, Appel LJ. *American Journal of Epidemiology.* 2009 Apr 1;169(7):893–900.

11. A randomized trial comparing a very low carbohydrate diet and a calorie-restricted low fat diet on body weight and cardiovascular risk factors in healthy women. Brehm BJ, Seeley RJ, Daniels SR, D'Alessio DA. *Journal of Clinical Endocrinology and Metabolism.* 2003 Apr;88(4):1617–23.

12. A randomized trial of a low-carbohydrate diet for obesity. Foster GD, Wyatt HR, Hill JO, McGuckin BG, Brill C, Mohammed BS, Szapary PO, Rader DJ, Edman JS, Klein S. *New England Journal of Medicine.* 2003 May 22;348(21):2082–90.

13. A reduced ratio of dietary carbohydrate to protein improves body composition and blood lipid profiles during weight loss in adult women. Layman DK, Boileau RA, Erickson DJ, Painter JE, Shiue H, Sather C, Christou DD. *Journal of Nutrition.* 2003 Feb;133(2):411–17.

14. Dietary protein and exercise have additive effects on body composition during weight loss in adult women. Layman DK, Evans E, Baum JI, Seyler J, Erickson DJ, Boileau RA. *Journal of Nutrition.* 2005 Aug;135(8):1903–10.

15. Carbohydrate restriction as the default treatment for type 2 diabetes and metabolic syndrome. Richard D. Feinman and Jeff S. Volek. *Scandinavian Cardiovascular Journal.* 2008 42:4, 256–63.

16. Adherence to a DASH-style diet and risk of coronary heart disease and stroke in women. Fung TT, Chiuve SE, McCullough ML, Rexrode KM, Logroscino G, Hu FB. *Archives of Internal Medicine.* 2008 Apr 14; 168(7):713-20. Erratum in: *Arch Intern Med.* 2008 Jun 23;168(12):1276.

17. Relation of consistency with the dietary approaches to stop hypertension diet and incidence of heart failure in men aged 45 to 79 years. Levitan EB, Wolk A, Mittleman MA. *American Journal of Cardiology.* 2009 Nov 15;104(10):1416–20.

18. Consistency with the DASH diet and incidence of heart failure. Levitan EB, Wolk A, Mittleman MA. *Archives of Internal Medicine.* 2009 May 11;169(9):851–57.

19. Diet-quality scores and the risk of type 2 diabetes in men. de Koning L, Chiuve SE, Fung TT, Willett WC, Rimm EB, Hu FB. *Diabetes Care.* 2011 May;34(5):1150–56.

20. Dietary patterns during adolescence and risk of type 2 diabetes in middle-aged women. Malik VS, Fung TT, van Dam RM, Rimm EB, Rosner B, Hu FB. *Diabetes Care.* 2012 Jan;35(1):12–18.

21. Association of dietary patterns with albuminuria and kidney function decline in older white women: a subgroup analysis from the Nurses' Health Study. Lin J, Fung TT, Hu FB, Curhan GC. *American Journal of Kidney Disease.* 2011 Feb;57(2):245–54.

22. DASH-style diet associates with reduced risk for kidney stones. Taylor EN, Fung TT, Curhan GC. *Journal of the American Society of Nephrology.* 2009 Oct;20(10):2253–59.

23. Low-carbohydrate diets, dietary approaches to stop hypertension–style diets, and the risk of postmenopausal breast cancer. Fung TT, Hu FB, Hankinson SE, Willett WC, Holmes MD. *American Journal of Epidemiology.* 2011 Sep 15;174(6):652–60. Epub 2011 Aug 10.

24. The Mediterranean and Dietary Approaches to Stop Hypertension (DASH) diets and colorectal cancer. Fung TT, Hu FB, Wu K, Chiuve SE, Fuchs CS, Giovannucci E. *American Journal of Clinical Nutrition.* 2010 Dec;92(6):1429–35.

25. DASH diet lowers blood pressure and lipid-induced oxidative stress in obesity. Lopes HF, Martin KL, Nashar K, Morrow JD, Goodfriend TL, Egan BM. *Hypertension.* 2003 Mar;41(3):422–30.

26. A dietary pattern that lowers oxidative stress increases antibodies to oxidized LDL: results from a randomized controlled feeding study. Miller ER 3rd, Erlinger TP, Sacks FM, Svetkey LP, Charleston J, Lin PH, Appel LJ. *Atherosclerosis.* 2005 Nov;183(1):175–82. Epub 2005 Apr 18.

27. The DASH diet may have beneficial effects on bone health. Doyle L, Cashman KD. *Nutrition Reviews.* 2004 May;62(5):215–20.

PART IV

Setting the Stage for Success

CHAPTER 14

Going to the Market, Going to Get Healthy

It can seem overwhelming to figure out which foods are healthy. There are incomprehensible Nutrition Fact labels. American Heart Association Heart-Checks. Claims of being a source of "whole grains" when there is very little actually in the product. Low fat. Reduced fat. And now grocery chains are getting into the fray with their own ideas of what makes healthy foods.

We are going to help you make sense of the food labels and health claims. Then, we will help you with building a grocery list and stocking up your kitchen to make it very easy to follow the DASH Diet Weight Loss Solution. Add in some recommendations for additional DASH-friendly recipes and favorite cookbooks, and you will be on track to be healthier for the rest of your life.

How to Make Sense of Food Labels, Check Marks, and Health Claims

Nutrition labels were developed to help people avoid less healthful foods, and choose foods with important nutrients. However, the net effect may have been to expect everyone to become a dietitian. Who travels to the grocery store with a calculator to see how each food fits into their daily plan?

Whenever I am asked what people should look for on the food labels, I always respond, "Choose mostly foods without labels." What on earth does that mean? Fresh fruits and vegetables don't have food labels. Some fresh fish, poultry, and meat don't have food labels. These are all unprocessed foods that happen to fit into a healthy diet. Going one step beyond this to include relatively unprocessed foods such as milk, yogurt, frozen vegetables and fruits without additives makes a great foundation for a healthy diet. It is more when you get into heavily processed foods (which we are not really recommending in this plan) that food labels become important.

Many of the alternative food "health" labels, such as check marks, can be confusing and may not correspond to the DASH recommendations. For example, some foods high in added sugars may have a health claim because they have added some whole grain. However, it probably is not something that you would choose to be part of your plan. This chapter will

Plain Yogurt

Nutrition Facts

8 servings per container

Serving size   2/3 cup (55g)

Amount per serving

Calories   230

	% Daily Value*
Total Fat 8g	**10%**
Saturated Fat 1g	**5%**
Trans Fat 0g	
Cholesterol 0mg	**0%**
Sodium 160mg	**7%**
Total Carbohydrate 37g	**13%**
Dietary Fiber 4g	**14%**
Total Sugars 12g	
Includes 10g Added Sugars	**20%**
Protein 3g	
Vitamin D 2mcg	10%
Calcium 260mg	20%
Iron 8mg	45%
Potassium 235mg	6%

* The % Daily Value (DV) tells you how much a nutrient in a serving of food contributes to a daily diet. 2,000 calories a day is used for general nutrition advice.

help you make great choices for healthy foods for the DASH Diet Weight Loss Solution.

In defense of the Nutrition Facts, many of the nutrients that are required on the labels can help people reduce their risk of developing or help manage some very common diseases and conditions, such as heart disease, hypertension, diabetes, and obesity. The key nutrients include calories, total fat, saturated fat, trans fats, cholesterol, sodium, total carbohydrates, and protein. And the vitamins and minerals on the labels are those of which people are most at risk for having deficiencies.

Specific information must be given on the Nutrition Facts panel label, as shown on page 150. In the following sections I will go through the panel, step-by-step, to explain the components.

Serving Size

First, you want to know how much is in a serving of the food. In this example (plain yogurt), the serving size is 1 cup, which is the amount in the entire container. If there are multiple servings in a container, the Nutrition Facts panel will help you see this. For example, a bag of microwave popcorn might contain two or three servings. You need to check to be sure what serving size the calories and nutrients are based on.

In general, for multiserving packages, there are standardized serving sizes. However, it gets a little confusing to compare single-serving containers of different sizes. For example, the standard serving of potato chips is 1 ounce. However, if you have a ½-ounce bag of chips, that is a serving for that package. For a 1½-ounce bag, the serving size for that package is the entire 1½ ounces, since it is assumed that you will consume the entire bag.

Cereals are one of the most challenging foods to judge a

serving size for. The standard serving size is 1 ounce by weight; however the volume can range from ¼ cup to 1¼ cups. And with some very dense cereals, such as Grape-Nuts, the label serving size is ½ cup, which is 2 ounces, or 2 DASH diet servings. It is very important to check the serving size and see how that compares with the serving size you want for the DASH Diet Weight Loss Solution.

Total Calories and Calories from Fat

Total calories are related to serving size. The calories from fat give you an idea of the nutrient density. Foods that are high in calories and without significant vitamins, minerals, or protein are considered to have a low nutrient density. They bring calories, but not much nutritional value. If someone eats a high-starch or high-fat diet, it is possible that he or she could be getting adequate calories, but still be malnourished. Because in the DASH Diet Weight Loss Solution we are really cutting back on refined starchy foods, you are less likely to have to worry about this problem. Real food tends to have more nutritional bang for the buck!

Nutrient Composition

The next section of the food label shows the grams of various nutrients in a serving, and the percent daily values. The daily values percentage can often be very confusing. Many people look at the percentage and think it represents the percent of the nutrient in the food. Using the yogurt example, the 4 grams of fat represent 6% of the requirement for a day, based on a 2,000-calorie diet. It doesn't mean that 6% of the calories in the yogurt come from fat. In fact, since 35 of the 150 calories come from fat (from the top section), 23% of the calories are from fat. (Okay, where is your calculator?) It is important for controlling cholesterol to choose foods that are low in saturated and trans fats. And our food recommendations in the DASH diet support that, without your having to spend too much time deciphering the labels, or needing that calculator.

Sodium and occasionally potassium are listed in this section. You, obviously, want to limit sodium and choose foods that are rich in potassium. However, again, many of the potassium-rich foods will not have food labels. Fish, meat, fruits, and vegetables are all great sources. Dairy foods will have a label, and they are also rich in potassium. Yes, they also contain naturally occurring sodium, but the net benefit is on the side of health with milk and yogurt. Most cheese is also high in added sodium, but you can find lower-sodium varieties, which are better choices. Salt is often added to speed ripening of the cheeses. Lower-sodium versions may have better taste, because they have ripened more slowly. Swiss cheese is naturally low-sodium, and if you choose the 2% milk version, it is reduced in saturated fat, as well.

In the carbohydrate section you will find total carbohydrates, fiber, and sugars. The carbohydrate that isn't sugar or fiber is mostly starch, which you can compute by subtracting fiber and sugar from the total carbohydrate value. Fiber content may also be broken down further to show grams of soluble fiber. And in the DASH Diet Weight Loss Solution, we definitely prefer whole grains and don't include much of the empty-calorie, refined starchy foods. So maybe we can avoid needing a calculator for this, too!

Additional vitamins and minerals with special health concerns are shown in the bottom section of the Nutrition Facts panel. Vitamin C, vitamin A, calcium, and iron content must be included on the label. Manufacturers may also list additional vitamins and minerals, if they choose. The calcium content (and vitamin D, if listed) is especially important if you are choosing nondairy substitutes. These products should have similar calcium, vitamin D, and protein as the dairy foods they are replacing.

Ingredients

Another requirement for food labels is that they must include an ingredient list. If you are concerned about cholesterol, you may want to go easy on foods that contain hydrogenated or partially hydrogenated fats. And now much of these ingredients have been replaced by coconut oil, palm oil, or palm kernel oil. We want to avoid these oils because they are very high in saturated fats. Since they tend to occur in processed, starchy foods, we should not see too much of them in your diet.

The ingredient list is another way to check how much sugar has been added to a food. Some of the many terms that indicate sugar include high fructose corn syrup, grape juice (and other fruit juices), agave, corn syrup, honey, molasses, dextrose, fructose, and lactose.

Since ingredients must be listed in order by weight (from the highest to the lowest), having many sources of sugar can help the manufacturer disguise the importance of sugar in the overall product formula. The Nutrition Facts panel will provide better information on the amount of sugar in a specific food. Many healthy DASH diet foods naturally contain sugars (such as fruits, yogurt, and milk) and should not be avoided, unless they contain added sugars. Again, read the ingredient list to see if sugars have been added, and compare calories for comparable foods. Choosing our new DASH diet foods, which are less processed, will naturally help you avoid the added sugars, without having to think about it too much.

Making Your List, to Make It Easy to Follow the Plan

In each section that introduced the phases of the DASH Diet Weight Loss Solution program, we had lists of foods to stock up on. It definitely makes it much easier to get on track and stay on track when you have all the right foods. It sets the stage for success. You will see yourself as being someone who can set goals and keep them, when you make it easier for yourself.

The key DASH diet foods are fruits, vegetables, low-fat and nonfat dairy, nuts and beans, lean meats, fish, and poultry. Keeping these foods on hand will make it easy to follow the program. If, on the other hand, you keep lots of candy, chips, cookies, and ice cream in your home, you will be inclined to fill up on the wrong foods. The foods in your kitchen and at work will determine what you eat. You want to make it easy to grab foods or make a last-minute meal that will keep you on track with the DASH diet.

Let's look at this from a family focus. Often, moms and dads keep lots of junk food around for the "kids." But then it is really the moms and dads who are eating most of the junk food, not the kids. Often I will suggest that people keep a tray of cut-up fresh fruits and veggies in the refrigerator to facilitate easy, healthy snacking. And then the parents say that it disappears before they get home from work. Yes, the kids will eat the healthy snacks if they are ready to eat. I'll give you another example. My sister-in-law would always fume when I brought fresh fruits and veggies to her Super Bowl parties. She is the type to load up on fatty, fried foods for the "special occasion." Her husband, on the other hand, continued to be amazed at how the kids ate up 100% of the fruits and vegetables, while trays of potato skins and Buffalo wings were still sitting on the table. If you serve healthy foods, they will eat. This is one of the collateral benefits of following this plan. It does make your whole family healthier.

Let's take it step-by-step.

Stock Up

You will want to stock your cupboards and refrigerator with staples that allow you to make a variety of meals without having to run to the store every day (unless, of course, you like to grocery shop daily). The lists below will provide a foundation for making it easy to follow this plan every day. If you don't have the right foods on hand, you will get off track very easily. But if you do have the key foods, this plan is easy to follow.

Making Great DASH Choices

Fruits and Vegetables

Fruits and vegetables are important sources of vitamin C, folate, potassium, and many other vitamins and minerals. The phytochemicals (*phyto-* means "plant") that produce color, scent, and flavor give special health benefits, improving certain health conditions and reducing the risk for many types of cancer. Fruits and vegetables have high water content, which makes them filling, while being low in calories. A small piece of fruit will typically have about 60 calories, primarily from fruit sugar. One-half cup of cooked nonstarchy vegetables will have about 25 calories. The starchy ones (primarily potatoes and winter squash) will have higher calories, about 60 per half-cup. Corn, which is starchy, is technically a grain, even though we eat it as if it were a vegetable. And it contains about 80 calories per half-cup.

Fruits and vegetables contain both soluble and nonsoluble fiber. As you may remember, soluble fiber is the type that soaks up fats and cholesterol in our digestive tract. Berries, plums, peaches, pears, and apples are some good sources. The nonsoluble fiber is "roughage," which is the type that makes us more "regular." Most fruits and vegetables are good sources. Both types of fiber are good for the digestive system. Fiber also slows down absorption of sugars during digestion, which can help to reduce the likelihood of blood sugar spikes, and helps us to feel satisfied longer after meals.

We have all heard that carrots are good for our eyes. But did you know that there are many types of health-promoting plant chemicals in fruits and vegetables? We don't want to bore you by getting too bogged down in the details, since our focus is on the whole foods rather than their parts. That said, many of the color-producing chemicals in food are antioxidants. Good examples include the carotenoids, such as beta-carotene, which make the orange color in carrots, and lycopene, which makes the red color in tomatoes. Anthocyananins are also strong antioxidants, and they make the red-purple-blue colors in foods. In general, the more colors on your plate, the healthier the meal. There really are only good choices here. Having a variety of vegetables and fruits at a meal helps to ensure that you are getting more types of nutrients and many health benefits.

Whole Grains

We all know that whole grains are healthier than the refined ones. During the refining process, many of the important vitamins and minerals are stripped away. Refined grains are enriched with some B vitamins and iron, but not with the same minerals or vitamins that were processed out of the grain. Most grains are wonderful sources of insoluble fiber, while oats and barley also have high amounts of soluble (functional) fiber.

One side note: If you bake with whole grain flour, store it somewhere cool or refrigerated. Whole grains are subject to rancidity, and therefore must be kept cold if not used quickly.

Nuts, Beans, and Seeds

Way back in the 1990s, when fat was "bad," we threw the baby out with the bathwater. Not all fats are problematic, and nuts and seeds are certainly wonderful sources of all kinds of nutrients, including heart-healthy fats. Add in the protein in nuts, and you also have a powerful tool to quench hunger. Nuts and seeds are rich in fiber, vitamins, and minerals such as potassium and magnesium.

Beans, of course, are rich in fiber, especially soluble fiber. They contain a little more starch than a serving of grain foods, about the amount of protein found in 1 ounce of cooked meat, little or no fat, and some important vitamins and minerals such as iron and zinc.

Low-Fat and Nonfat Dairy

Dairy is one of the key DASH diet foods. When the first study was done, one of the three test groups had a diet with extra amounts of fruits and vegetables, without adding in extra dairy. They did not see the blood pressure–lowering effect of the full DASH plan. The main problem with dairy has been the butterfat, which is very rich in saturated fats. Saturated fat is associated with increased risk for diabetes and inflammation, and forms the raw material for making cholesterol. Choosing reduced-fat, low-fat, and nonfat dairy will help to avoid the problems. Your best choices are nonfat milk and yogurt, and cheeses that are made from 2% milk or are low-fat. I have met a few people who actually like fat-free cheese, but if you are not one of them, choose the 2% cheeses.

When buying cheese, choose reduced-fat or nonfat varieties. When you are dining out, you generally don't have a low-fat cheese option available, so have it at home whenever you can. And cheeses are very low in lactose.

Nonfat yogurt is especially good. If you are watching calories, choose yogurts with little or no added sugar. The labels on yogurt can be confusing as to sugar content because of the milk sugar. (And you should note that most of the milk sugar has been converted to lactic acid in yogurts, although the label does not reflect this.) Choose yogurts with less than 120 calories for a 6- to 8-ounce serving. As an added benefit, most people with lactose intolerance can handle yogurt very well. If you are sensitive to lactose or milk proteins, you can choose dairy substitutes. Take care to choose products with calcium and vitamin D that are equal to their real dairy counterparts.

If you are lactose-intolerant, you can find lactose-free milk, or take lactose digesting enzymes to reduce the lactose. And cheeses and yogurt tend to be very low in lactose. See Appendix A for more information.

Which is better, butter or margarine? A soft margarine that doesn't contain trans fats is your best choice. Another good selection criteria is to look for margarines with plant stanols or sterols, such as Smart Balance. The stanols help to reduce cholesterol levels, which can be an added benefit. For special baking or cooking, you can occasionally use butter, as long as you use it rarely and in small quantities. I choose butter for special meals for its flavor, but I rarely use either margarine or butter as part of my routine diet.

Lean Meats, Fish, and Poultry

For the nonvegetarians, lean meats, fish, and poultry can be great protein sources, as long as we do not choose the ones high in saturated fats or added sodium.

When the relationship between heart disease and cholesterol was first uncovered, everyone told us to lower our intake of red meat and high-fat dairy foods. People replaced the dairy with soda, which was a very poor idea for any reason, but especially for bone health. And people cut back on red meat, but then became tired of having the "same old chicken again." The great news is that today we don't have to cut back, because there are healthier options. We can include red meat and dairy foods that are low in fat, along with poultry, fish, and vegetable protein sources.

When choosing beef or pork, look for cuts that include the terms "loin" or "round" in their names. Sirloin, tenderloin, and loin chops (including New York strip steaks) are all lean cuts. Pork tenderloin is even lower in fat and calories than a boneless, skinless chicken breast. Choose meats that are graded "select" and only occasionally have "choice" or "prime," which are much higher in fat. And of course, the fat in meats is high in saturated fat. Since restaurants tend to serve choice or prime cuts, seafood can be a better choice when eating out (assuming the seafood isn't swimming in butter). And of course, skinless chicken and turkey are low in saturated fat.

For ground beef, 95% lean ground sirloin is a perfect choice and is just slightly higher in fat and calories than a chicken breast. There will be little or no fat to pour off, which is a very good sign. Watch out if you are buying ground chicken or turkey. Often skin and fat are added, which will make these choices much higher in saturated fat than lean beef.

Dark poultry meat is becoming popular again, because it is

more flavorful and tender than white meat. And it is much higher in monounsaturated fats than in saturated fat, so chicken thighs and legs can be a high-flavor addition to your poultry choices.

Seafood is mostly very low in fat, and most of it that is high-fat has extremely healthy fats, the omega-3s. Good examples include salmon, tuna, sardines, and swordfish. The low-fat seafood, including shrimp and other crustaceans, is very low in calories and is a great way to add variety to your meals. Surprisingly, even shellfish that may be high in cholesterol can be a heart-healthy choice, since it is so very low in total fat and virtually free of saturated fat. Even fatty fish are still in the lean range when compared to meat and poultry.

In addition to proteins and fat, lean animal foods are great sources of many additional nutrients, such as vitamins and minerals. For example, beef is very rich in zinc, vitamins B12 and B6, and iron.

Heart-Healthy Fats

The fats that we would like to have in our diets include the monounsaturated fats and the special long-chain polyunsaturated fats known as the omega-3 fatty acids (found in some nuts and fish). The fats that we want to go easy on include the saturated and trans fats and, surprisingly, most of the polyunsaturated fats.

We know that saturated fat is associated with increased production of cholesterol, but it is less well known that excess carbs tend to exacerbate this. So the DASH Diet Weight Loss Solution will help keep cholesterol under control by impacting both factors. When the recommendation to reduce saturated fat first came out, it was accompanied by a recommendation to replace it with polyunsaturated fats, such as those from corn oil or soybean oil. Now these oils, which are rich in omega-6 fatty acids, are considered to be less healthy in high amounts. The omega-6 fats are associated with increased risk of heart disease, depression, autoimmune diseases, and inflammation. The beneficial monounsaturated fats, found in olive oil and canola oil, are associated with lower rates of heart disease and some types of cancer, as are the omega-3 fats found in seafood and some kinds of nuts, such as walnuts.

Heart-healthy choices include olive oil, canola oil, peanut oil, and to a lesser extent, corn, soy, and safflower oil. Peanut oil is a great choice for cooking at high temperatures, such as stir frying, since it is rich in monounsaturated fats but has a higher smoke point than olive oil. That is, it will tolerate higher cooking temperatures without giving off the toxic smoke of oils with lower smoke points.

Coconut oil, palm oil, and palm kernel oil are vegetable sources of saturated fat. Coconut oil may be found in popcorn, especially commercially prepared fresh popcorn. And all these fats are now often found in cookies, crackers, and other pastries and baked goods, where they have replaced much of the trans fats. Even though many manufacturers have removed them, you still need to watch out for and avoid hydrogenated or partially hydrogenated fats, which are the sources of trans fats.

Foods for Your Grocery List

The following are some suggestions to help you stock your kitchen with DASH-friendly foods:

Canned, Bottled, and Dry Foods

- Diced tomatoes, no added salt
- Tomato sauce, no added salt
- Tomato paste, no added salt
- Kidney beans, no added salt
- Black beans, no added salt
- Lentils

- Canned tuna, in water, low-salt
- Canned salmon, low-salt
- Canned chicken, low-salt
- Extra virgin olive oil
- Peanut oil
- Canola oil
- Salad dressings
- Mustard
- Oatmeal, unsweetened
- High-fiber cereals without added sugar
- Whole wheat bread, including "light" or "lite" kinds
- Nuts, preferably unsalted

Spices and Herbs

- Bag of onions
- Bulbs of garlic
- Shallots
- Fresh herbs
- Dry spices including basil, oregano, parsley flakes, thyme, marjoram, paprika, rosemary, ginger, poultry seasoning, sage, onion powder, garlic powder, chili powder, etc.
- Salt substitutes, including lemon-pepper

Frozen

- Individual and mixed vegetables, without sauces
- Sliced pepper and onion mix
- Diced onions
- Diced green peppers
- Frozen skinless boneless chicken breasts
- Frozen 95% lean ground sirloin (and patties)
- Frozen yogurt, with no added sugar
- Frozen fruit

Refrigerated

- Lemon juice
- Lime juice
- Sliced deli meats, low-sodium
- Cheese, low-sodium and reduced-fat

Fresh from the Market (Don't forget farmers' markets!)

- Lettuces and other greens
- Carrots, baby, sliced or grated
- Grape or cherry tomatoes or other high-flavor tomatoes
- Coleslaw mix
- Broccoli slaw
- Radishes
- Peppers
- Broccoli
- Cauliflower
- Red cabbage
- Cucumber
- Beets
- Fresh fruit

Meat Counter

- Fresh fish (See table on pages 168–69.)
- Lean meat and poultry (See tables on pages 166–67.)

Dairy

- Low-fat or nonfat, low-sodium cheeses: cheddar, Swiss, Colby-Jack, mozzarella; sliced and grated
- Light individually packaged cheeses such as Mini Baby-bel Light, The Laughing Cow Light Wedges, string cheese, Kraft 2% Singles, and 2% or 1% cottage cheese

- Nonfat yogurt, artificially sweetened
- Skim milk
- Egg substitutes
- Eggs or omega-3-rich eggs

Equipment

Having the right equipment will make your life easier, whether you like to cook or don't want to spend your time cooking.

- Countertop grill. This allows the quick preparation of lean meats, fish, and poultry. The newer versions have removable grill surfaces for easy cleanup.
- Toaster oven. Great for making small meals or reheating certain leftovers.
- Microwave. Always great for reheating or making quick scrambled eggs.
- Blender. Can help with pureeing vegetables to sneak into sauces or soups, in addition to making great smoothies.
- Digital kitchen scale. Helps make it easy to avoid "portion distortion."
- Food processor. Makes it a breeze to cut up vegetables.
- Mandoline or V-slicer. For quickly cut up veggies. Even faster than a food processor, with less cleanup.
- Instant-read digital thermometer. Tells you when your meat is cooked correctly, and when your leftovers are heated enough (165°).
- Great super-sharp knives, not serrated. Make cutting up vegetables easier. Thinner blades are easier to push through larger vegetables.

Making Great Choices for Meat, Poultry, and Fish

Calories and Fat in 3 Ounces of Cooked Lean Beef

	Calories	Fat (g)	Saturated fat (g)	Cholesterol (mg)
Top round roast, broiled	153	4.2	1.4	71
Eye-round, roasted	143	4.2	1.5	59
Shoulder pot roast, roasted	136	4.7	1.6	54
Round tip roast, roasted	147	5.7	1.8	60
Shoulder steak, braised	161	6.0	1.9	80
Top sirloin steak, broiled	166	6.1	2.4	76
Bottom round, roasted	161	6.3	2.1	66
Top loin steak, broiled	176	8.0	3.1	65
Tenderloin steak, broiled	175	8.1	3.0	71
T-bone steak, broiled	172	8.2	3.0	48
Tri-tip roast, roasted	177	8.2	3.0	70
NY strip steak, broiled	161	6.0	2.3	56
Ground beef, 95% lean, pan-broiled	139	5.0	2.2	65
Ground beef, 90% lean, pan-broiled	173	9.1	3.7	70
Ground beef, 85% lean, pan-broiled	197	11.9	4.7	73

Calories and Fat in 3 Ounces of Cooked Lean Pork

	Calories	Fat (g)	Saturated fat (g)	Cholesterol (mg)
Pork tenderloin, roasted	140	4	1	65
Pork top loin roast, roasted	170	6	2	65
Pork top loin chop, broiled	170	7	2	70
Pork loin center chop, broiled	170	7	3	70
Pork sirloin roast, roasted	180	9	3	75
Ham, lean, roasted	145	5.5	1.8	53

Calories and Fat in 3 Ounces of Cooked Lean Poultry

	Calories	Fat (g)	Saturated fat (g)	Cholesterol (mg)
Chicken breast, with skin, roasted	167	6.6	1.9	71
Chicken breast, skinless, roasted	140	3.0	0.9	72
Chicken thigh, with skin, roasted	210	13.2	3.7	79
Chicken thigh, skinless, roasted	178	9.2	2.6	81
Turkey breast, skinless, roasted	115	0.6	0.2	71
Turkey whole, with skin, roasted	146	4.9	1.4	89
Ground turkey, cooked	200	11.2	2.9	87
Ground turkey breast, cooked	98	3.8	1.0	44

Calories and Fat in 3 Ounces of Cooked Fish and Seafood

	Calories	Fat (g)	Saturated fat (g)	Cholesterol (mg)
Blue crab	100	1	0	90
Catfish	140	9	2	50
Clams (about 12 small)	100	1.5	0	55
Cod	90	0.5	0	45
Flounder/sole	100	1.5	0.5	60
Haddock	100	1	0	80
Halibut	110	2	0	35
Lobster	80	0	0	60
Mackerel	210	13	1.5	60
Ocean perch	110	2	0	50
Orange roughy	80	1	0	20
Oysters (about 12 medium)	100	3.5	1	115
Pollock	90	1	0	80
Rainbow trout	140	6	2	60
Rockfish	100	2	0	40
Salmon, Atlantic/coho	160	7	1	50
Salmon, chum/pink	130	4	1	70
Salmon, sockeye	180	9	1.5	75
Scallops (6 large, 14 small)	120	1	0	55
Shrimp	80	1	0	165
Swordfish	130	4.5	1	40
Tuna, canned in water	116	0.8	0.2	30
White fish	172	7.5	1.2	77

Omega-3 Fatty Acid Content in Fish and Seafood

	EPA, grams	DHA, grams
Cod liver oil (1 tablespoon)	1.0	1.5
Mackerel (3.5 ounces)	0.9	1.4
Salmon (3.5 ounces)	0.8	0.6
Herring (3.5 ounces)	0.7	0.9
Anchovy (3.5 ounces)	0.5	0.9
Tuna (3.5 ounces)	0.3	0.9
Blue fish (3.5 ounces)	0.2	0.5
Swordfish (3.5 ounces)	0.1	0.5

EPA = eicosapentaenoic acid, DHA = docosahexenoic acid

CHAPTER 15

Making the DASH Diet Your Habit

A recent study showed that making one good habit could lead to adding other healthy habits without much thought about it. For weight loss, it was more effective for people to track what they were eating than for a doctor to browbeat them into eating better. Why did that work? Because when people started tracking what they were eating, they became more aware of their actions.

So what would be great for helping to adopt the DASH Diet Weight Loss Solution behaviors? Tracking. Keeping track of your actions. This will lead to more self-awareness. If you eat poorly, and the next day your weight and your blood pressure are up, maybe there is a connection. But you will be the one making that connection. Not anyone else.

[I have one more secret habit that will be key to your diet change. Make half your plate veggies. Nonstarchy veggies. As simple as that.]

All through this book we have indicated specific changes for you to make to adopt the DASH Diet Weight Loss Solution to help you reach and maintain a healthy weight. It is helpful to track your food intake, exercise, and weight to see how your actions pay off in terms of making you healthier. Larger copies of all the forms provided here are available on our website at http://dashdiet.org/forms. You can download them as many times as you want, to continue to track your progress.

In this book we have two different types of forms for tracking your food intake. One counts food groups, and the other is more of a pictorial way of representing your meal plans. Choose the form that seems most useful for you. There is a food group tracker for Phase 1 and Phase 2.

We also have forms to track exercise, weight, blood pressure, blood sugar (if you need to), and overall health and well-being. The blood pressure and blood sugar logs allow you to track how you are responding to the program. These will be useful for your physician, especially if the numbers are trending toward the low side, or are reliably in the normal range. Both the blood pressure and the sugar readings are immediate health indicators. You don't have to take these readings unless you have been instructed to do so by your physician.

On the first line, write in your typical blood pressure readings before starting the plan. Hopefully, your blood pressure will improve as you change your eating style, lose weight, and add exercise. As a reminder, if your blood pressure is 140/90, 140 is the systolic reading and 90 is the diastolic reading.

The DASH Diet Food Group Servings Check Off Form for Phase 1

Food Groups	Monday	Tuesday	Wednesday	Thursday	Friday	Saturday	Sunday
Grains, starches, sweets None in Phase 1							
Fruits None in Phase 1							
Vegetables ½ cup cooked vegetables, 1 cup leafy greens, 1 cup raw, 6 oz vegetable	☐☐☐☐☐☐	☐☐☐☐☐☐	☐☐☐☐☐☐	☐☐☐☐☐☐	☐☐☐☐☐☐	☐☐☐☐☐☐	☐☐☐☐☐☐
Low-fat dairy (preferably) 1–2 oz skim or low-fat milk in coffee, 6–8 oz yogurt, 1 oz cheese, ½ cup cottage cheese	☐☐☐☐	☐☐☐☐	☐☐☐☐	☐☐☐☐	☐☐☐☐	☐☐☐☐	☐☐☐☐
Beans, nuts, seeds ¼ cup beans, nuts, seeds, 2 T peanut butter	☐☐☐☐	☐☐☐☐	☐☐☐☐	☐☐☐☐	☐☐☐☐	☐☐☐☐	☐☐☐☐
Lean meat, fish, poultry, eggs, soy meat substitutes (after cooking) Each ☐ = 1 oz 1 egg = 1 oz, 2 egg whites = 1 oz	☐☐☐☐☐ ☐☐☐☐☐	☐☐☐☐☐ ☐☐☐☐☐	☐☐☐☐☐ ☐☐☐☐☐	☐☐☐☐☐ ☐☐☐	☐☐☐☐☐ ☐☐☐	☐☐☐☐☐ ☐☐☐	☐☐☐☐☐ ☐☐☐
Fats, fatty sauces 1 T salad dressing 1 t butter, oil	☐☐☐☐☐☐	☐☐☐☐☐☐	☐☐☐☐☐☐	☐☐☐☐☐☐	☐☐☐☐☐☐	☐☐☐☐☐☐	☐☐☐☐☐☐
Water, liquids 8 oz	☐☐☐☐☐☐ ☐☐☐☐☐☐	☐☐☐☐☐☐ ☐☐☐☐☐☐	☐☐☐☐☐☐ ☐☐☐☐☐☐	☐☐☐☐☐☐ ☐☐☐☐☐☐	☐☐☐☐☐☐ ☐☐☐☐☐☐	☐☐☐☐☐☐ ☐☐☐☐☐☐	☐☐☐☐☐☐ ☐☐☐☐☐☐
Alcohol None in Phase 1							
Exercise (each ☐ = 10 minutes)	☐☐☐☐☐ ☐☐☐☐☐	☐☐☐☐☐ ☐☐☐☐☐	☐☐☐☐☐ ☐☐☐☐☐	☐☐☐☐ ☐☐☐☐	☐☐☐☐ ☐☐☐☐	☐☐☐☐ ☐☐☐☐	☐☐☐☐ ☐☐☐☐

Grains, starches _____   Vegetables _____   Dairy _____   Fats _____

Fruits _____   Beans, nuts _____   Lean meats _____   Fluid _____

Alcohol _____   Exercise _____

The DASH Diet Food Group Servings Check Off Form for Phase 2

Food Groups	Monday	Tuesday	Wednesday	Thursday	Friday	Saturday	Sunday
Grains, starches, sweets 1 slice bread; ½ cup cooked pasta, rice; ½ cup cooked cereal, corn, potatoes; ¼ bagel; 1 oz dry cereal; ½ English muffin, bun; 2 cups popcorn; 2 small cookies	☐☐☐☐☐☐ ☐☐	☐☐☐☐☐☐ ☐☐	☐☐☐☐☐☐ ☐☐	☐☐☐☐☐☐ ☐☐	☐☐☐☐☐☐ ☐☐	☐☐☐☐☐☐ ☐☐	☐☐☐☐☐☐ ☐☐
Fruits 4 oz juice, small fruit, ¼ cup dried fruit, ½ cup canned fruit, 1 cup diced raw fruit	☐☐☐☐☐	☐☐☐☐☐	☐☐☐☐☐	☐☐☐☐☐	☐☐☐☐☐	☐☐☐☐☐	☐☐☐☐☐
Vegetables ½ cup cooked vegetables, 1 cup leafy greens, 6 oz vegetable juice	☐☐☐☐☐☐	☐☐☐☐☐☐	☐☐☐☐☐☐	☐☐☐☐☐☐	☐☐☐☐☐☐	☐☐☐☐☐☐	☐☐☐☐☐☐
Low-fat dairy 8 oz skim or low-fat milk, 8 oz low-fat/fat-free yogurt, 1 oz reduced-fat cheese, ½ cup fat-free or low-fat cottage cheese	☐☐☐☐	☐☐☐☐	☐☐☐☐	☐☐☐☐	☐☐☐☐	☐☐☐☐	☐☐☐☐
Beans, nuts, seeds ¼ cup beans, nuts, seeds, 2 T peanut butter	☐☐☐☐	☐☐☐☐	☐☐☐☐	☐☐☐☐	☐☐☐☐	☐☐☐☐	☐☐☐☐
Lean meat, fish, poultry, eggs, soy meat substitutes (after cooking) Each ☐ = 1 oz 1 egg = 1 oz, 2 egg whites = 1 oz	☐☐☐☐☐ ☐☐☐☐☐	☐☐☐☐☐ ☐☐☐☐☐	☐☐☐☐☐ ☐☐☐☐☐	☐☐☐☐☐ ☐☐☐☐☐	☐☐☐☐☐ ☐☐☐☐☐	☐☐☐☐☐ ☐☐☐☐☐	☐☐☐☐☐ ☐☐☐☐☐
Fats, fatty sauces 1 T salad dressing 1 t butter, oil	☐☐☐☐☐☐	☐☐☐☐☐☐	☐☐☐☐☐☐	☐☐☐☐☐☐	☐☐☐☐☐☐	☐☐☐☐☐☐	☐☐☐☐☐☐
Water, liquids 8 oz	☐☐☐☐☐ ☐☐☐☐☐	☐☐☐☐☐ ☐☐☐☐☐	☐☐☐☐☐ ☐☐☐☐☐	☐☐☐☐☐ ☐☐☐☐☐	☐☐☐☐☐ ☐☐☐☐☐	☐☐☐☐☐ ☐☐☐☐☐	☐☐☐☐☐ ☐☐☐☐☐
Alcohol 1 oz liquor, 3 oz wine, 12 oz beer	☐☐	☐☐	☐☐	☐☐	☐☐	☐☐	☐☐
Exercise (each ☐ = 10 minutes)	☐☐☐☐☐ ☐☐☐☐☐	☐☐☐☐☐ ☐☐☐☐☐	☐☐☐☐☐ ☐☐☐☐☐	☐☐☐☐☐ ☐☐☐☐☐	☐☐☐☐☐ ☐☐☐☐☐	☐☐☐☐☐ ☐☐☐☐☐	☐☐☐☐☐ ☐☐☐☐☐

Grains, starches _____   Vegetables _____   Fats _____
Fruits _____   Beans, nuts _____   Fluid _____
Alcohol _____   Exercise _____
Dairy _____   Lean meats _____

The Daily Meal Plan Tracker

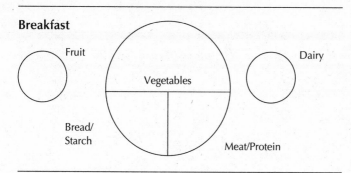

Breakfast

Fruit

Vegetables

Dairy

Bread/
Starch

Meat/Protein

Snack

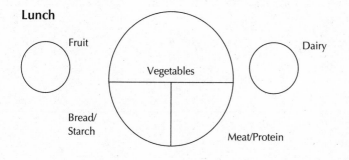

Lunch

Fruit

Vegetables

Dairy

Bread/
Starch

Meat/Protein

Snack

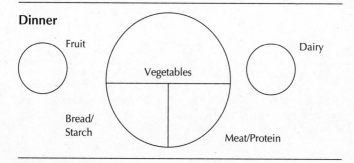

Dinner

Fruit

Vegetables

Dairy

Bread/
Starch

Meat/Protein

Other Snack:

Activities:

Blood Pressure Log

	Systolic (top reading)	Diastolic (bottom reading)
Day 1		
Day 2		
Day 3		
Day 4		
Day 5		
Day 6		
Day 7		
Day 8		
Day 9		
Day 10		
Day 11		
Day 12		
Day 13		
Day 14		
Day 15		
Day 16		
Day 17		
Day 18		
Day 19		
Day 20		
Day 21		

Use the exercise log to monitor the activity you perform. Remember, set a goal of doing something active every day. If you can't do 30 or more minutes at one time, schedule three or more 10-minute sessions.

Weekly Exercise Log

	Type of Activity	Time	How do I feel?
Day 1			
Day 2			
Day 3			
Day 4			
Day 5			
Day 6			
Day 7			

Getting to a healthier weight or maintaining a healthy weight is a key goal for getting healthier. The following form will provide a convenient way to keep track of your progress with weight control and your waistline.

Weight Log

	Weight	Waist size
Goal weight		
Initial weight		
Week 1		
Week 2		
Week 3		

(Continued)

	Weight	Waist size
Week 4		
Week 5		
Week 6		
Week 7		
Week 8		

Additional benefits of making changes in diet, weight, and activity are improved mood, higher energy level, and enhanced sense of control over your health. A diary of your feelings may provide you with additional information that will help you sustain your behavior changes. The following is a model for a simple diary to track how the DASH Diet Weight Loss Solution is affecting your life.

Overall DASH Diet Outcome Log

	Mood, energy level, self-confidence, etc.
Initial	
Week 1	
Week 2	
Week 3	
Week 4	
Month 2	
Month 3	

Overall DASH Diet Outcome Log

Mood, energy level, self-confidence, etc.

Month 4

Month 5

Month 6

As mentioned above, all these forms are available for downloading in larger formats at http://dashdiet.org/forms.

CHAPTER 16

Super-Simple, Fabulous Recipes to Make the DASH Diet Your Own

We have created a variety of recipes to make it easy for you to prepare healthy dishes at home. They mostly have short preparation time, but the ones that do take longer to prepare generally make enough for several meals. Weekends are the times to make dishes that will last for several days.

Beef and Pork

Marla's Barbecue with Shredded Beef
Mexican Meatloaf
No Crust Pizza
Mexican-Spiced Pork Chops
Meaty Sauce over Spaghetti Squash
Hearty Extra Veggie Chili
Grilled Steak Salad
Super-Savory Sliders

Taco Salad
The World's Best Meatloaf
Mango-Berry Salsa with Grilled Pork Loin

Marla's Barbecue with Shredded Beef

3 pounds beef stew meat, cut into 1-inch chunks
¼ cup water
1 large (28-ounce) can tomato sauce
1 cup diced onions (fresh or ½ cup frozen)
1 cup diced yellow bell pepper
3 cloves garlic, minced
¼ cup brown sugar
½ cup orange juice
¼ cup yellow mustard (not dry)
¼ cup red wine vinegar
1 tablespoon Worcestershire sauce
⅛ teaspoon chili powder
⅛ teaspoon cayenne pepper
⅛ teaspoon black pepper

I use a pressure cooker, to speed up cooking the beef, adding about ¼ cup water to the bottom. My pressure cooker doesn't have a pressure gauge. If yours does, keep pressure at about 150 pounds. Cook while under pressure for about 20 minutes. I remove the cooker from the heat, and allow the pressure to drop naturally as it cools. You could also braise the beef slowly, on low heat, on top of the stove with the tomato sauce for several hours, or until fork tender.

After cooking, reserve any remaining cooking liquid. Shred the beef using two forks; remove any large pieces of fat or connective tissue. Return to the pressure cooker (or a large skillet or saucepan). Add the onions, peppers, and garlic, and simmer gently with some of the reserved cooking liquid. When the onions and peppers are soft, add the rest of the cooking liquid, tomato sauce, brown sugar, orange juice, mustard, and vinegar. You can take your time doing this, and allow the mixture to simmer gently and develop more flavors. If you prefer a sweeter barbecue sauce you can add a little extra brown sugar. Then add the Worcestershire sauce, chili powder, cayenne pepper, and black pepper. Allow to simmer for another 30 minutes, or longer if that fits your schedule.

Serve on buns for your family members who aren't reducing starches, or serve directly on the plate. Top with cheese, if desired.

Makes about 12 servings.

Hints: Freeze about half the leftovers for enjoying later. Refrigerate the rest for another meal, two to three days later.

You can also add Tabasco sauce or other hot sauce to make this spicier.

When making without a pressure cooker, first brown the meat at medium temperature with the onions, peppers, and garlic, then add the tomato sauce and reduce the temperature to low. You can add the additional ingredients later, as the meat starts to soften.

Great side dishes for this include applesauce, sweet corn, and coleslaw.

Mexican Meatloaf

2 tablespoons olive oil
½ cup diced onion
1 medium carrot, diced or thickly grated
1 stalk celery, diced
1 garlic clove, minced
1 pound ground beef
6 ounces soft Mexican chorizo, removed from casing and
   crumbled
2 jalapeño peppers, diced
¾ teaspoon salt
¼ teaspoon freshly ground black pepper
¼ teaspoon cayenne pepper
½ teaspoon ground cumin
2 eggs, well beaten
½ cup unseasoned bread crumbs

Preheat oven to 375°F.

In a skillet, heat the oil over medium-high heat. Add the onion, carrot, celery, and garlic. Cook, stirring often, until vegetables are soft, about 8 minutes. Set aside until cool enough to handle.

In a large bowl combine the sautéed vegetables, ground beef, chorizo, and diced jalapeños.

In a medium bowl, combine the salt, pepper, cayenne, cumin, and eggs. Mix well with a fork and pour it on top of the mixed meats. Add the bread crumbs and mix thoroughly with clean hands. (You may want to remove your rings first.)

Put the mixture into a 9-by-13-inch loaf pan and insert a meat thermometer into the center. Bake 40–45 minutes, or until the interior temperature is 160°F. Remove from the oven and carefully pour off any accumulated pan juices.

Makes about 10 servings.

Hint: We use a special meatloaf pan, with an inner slotted pan that fits into an outer pan. This allows the fat from the meatloaf to drip into the outer pan. You will also want to place the meatloaf pan on a baking sheet in the oven, to prevent drips and spills.

No Crust Pizza

1 pound extra-lean ground sirloin
1 medium onion, thinly sliced
1 or 2 red, yellow, or orange peppers, sliced
2 cloves garlic, minced
1 14.5-ounce can diced tomatoes, no salt added
Italian seasonings
8 ounces shredded 2% mozzarella cheese

Preheat the oven to 425°F.

Heat a large nonstick skillet over medium-high heat. Add the ground beef, cook 3 minutes, turn down heat to medium. Add the onions, peppers, and garlic. Continue cooking about 5 more minutes, or until the beef is thoroughly browned and the onions are soft.

Add the tomatoes and seasonings, and cook another 8–10 minutes to thicken the sauce.

Place the ground beef mixture on the bottom of a large shallow glassware dish (such as a Corningware 1½-quart oval or round baking dish). Top with the shredded mozzarella cheese, and bake in the oven for 20–25 minutes, or until slightly browned.

Makes 6–8 servings.

Hints: You can add any additional vegetables that you like, such as mushrooms, sliced tomatoes, artichoke hearts, zucchini, yellow squash, etc. You could also bake in the skillet, if it is oven-safe; that is, it has a metal handle and no plastic parts.

Mexican-Spiced Pork Chops

4 butterfly cut loin pork chops (2 pounds)
1 tablespoon canola oil

Spice Rub Mixture

2 tablespoons paprika
2 tablespoons chili powder
2 tablespoons brown sugar or Splenda Brown Sugar Blend
1 tablespoon ground cumin
1 tablespoon ground black pepper
1 tablespoon ground white pepper
1–2 teaspoons ground cayenne pepper
1 teaspoon ground cinnamon
½ teaspoon salt

Mix all the ingredients for the spice rub.

Dredge the pork chops through the spices, coating both sides. Pre-heat the oil in a skillet on medium-high heat. Place the pork chops in the skillet, reduce heat to medium, and cook about 4 minutes on each side, until well browned.

Makes 4 servings.

Hint: Great side dishes include applesauce, our Mango-Melon Salsa,* or other fruit salsas or chutneys.

Meaty Sauce over Spaghetti Squash

1 pound extra-lean ground sirloin (could substitute lean ground turkey)
½ medium onion, diced, or ½ cup frozen onions
2 cloves garlic, crushed or minced
1 14.5-ounce can diced tomatoes, no added salt
1 14.5-ounce can tomato sauce, no added salt

½ teaspoon dry
   Italian seasonings
1 medium spaghetti squash
4 fresh basil leaves cut into thin strips

Preheat the oven to 375°F.

Brown the ground beef in a nonstick skillet over medium heat. Add the diced onions directly to the cooking ground beef, to sauté. Before adding the garlic, turn the heat down slightly. Then add the garlic. (Hint: Remove the skin by smashing it under the blade of a chef's knife. You can either mince the garlic or squeeze it through a garlic press.)

After the meat is fully browned and the onions are mostly translucent, add the diced tomatoes and tomato sauce. Then add Italian seasonings to your own taste. Turn down the heat to low, and allow to simmer and thicken.

Now for the spaghetti squash. Cut the squash in half first, and scrape out the seeds. Boil in a large pot for 30 minutes, or fill a rectangular baking dish partway with water, place the squash halves with the rind facing up, and bake for about 40 minutes, or until soft.

Add the basil to the spaghetti sauce.

Then, pick up the squash lining just like you would pasta. Top with the spaghetti sauce, and enjoy.

Makes 4 servings.

Hints: Add a wonderful salad, and you have a low-calorie meal with about 5 servings of vegetables and 3 ounces of lean meat.

To make this a vegetarian dish, add soy-based crumbles instead of the sirloin. Use 1 tablespoon of olive oil to sauté the onions and garlic before adding the crumbles. Keep the temperature slightly less than medium, to avoid burning the garlic, which would create a harsh flavor.

If you have leftover spaghetti sauce, freeze for another use.

Hearty Extra Veggie Chili

1 pound extra-lean ground sirloin
1 medium onion, diced (or 1 cup frozen diced onions)
1 cup pepper strips (fresh or frozen)
2 cloves garlic, minced
1 14.5-ounce can diced tomatoes, no added salt
1 15-ounce can tomato sauce, no added salt
1 15.5-ounce can black beans, low-salt
1 15.5-ounce can kidney beans, low-salt
2 tablespoons chili powder
2 tablespoons paprika
1 teaspoon ground black pepper
½ bag frozen carrots, cauliflower, and broccoli

Heat a large nonstick skillet over medium-high heat. Add the ground beef, onions, and peppers, cook 3 minutes, and turn down the heat to medium. Stir occasionally while continuing to cook. Turn down the heat to medium-low and add the garlic. (Higher temperatures cause the garlic to turn bitter.) Continue to cook about 3 more minutes or until the meat is thoroughly browned.

Add the tomatoes, beans, and seasonings. Mix well, and allow to simmer for about 5 minutes. Then add the frozen vegetables. Continue to simmer for 30–60 minutes. If the chili starts to get really thick, you could add water or some tomato sauce.

Makes about 10 1-cup servings.

Hints: To make this a vegetarian dish, eliminate the beef entirely or replace with soy-based crumbles.

You could use lean ground turkey instead of the beef.

This chili is a wonderful quick meal solution. And it is almost impossible to overeat, since it is so packed with veggies.

Grilled Steak Salad

2 boneless New York strip steaks (about 10 ounces each)
1 garlic clove, cut in half
salt-free steak seasoning (or mix your own with 1 teaspoon each of ground black pepper, paprika, garlic powder, onion powder, cayenne pepper, and ¼ teaspoon coriander)
4 cups romaine lettuce, cut into 1-inch-wide strips or baby field greens
2 ripe pears, sliced
blue cheese crumbles (optional)
French vinaigrette dressing

Pat the steaks dry with a paper towel. Rub with the cut garlic clove. Then dredge through the seasoning mix. (Discard the seasoning mix after using.) Grill the steaks over medium-high heat about 5 minutes per side, or until your preferred degree of doneness.

Slice the steaks into ½-inch-wide strips. Place on top of the lettuce; add pear slices and optional blue cheese, and dress with the French vinaigrette.

Makes 4 servings.

Super-Savory Sliders

These sliders are very high flavor. Unfortunately, they come without a bun. (You know the drill.) But they will make a really satisfying main course for your dinner.

1 tablespoon olive or canola oil
½ large Bermuda onion or 1 medium, sliced very thin
1 small pat of butter
¼ cup red wine
1 pound extra-lean ground sirloin
4 slices 2% Swiss cheese
2 cups grape tomatoes

Preheat the oil in a nonstick skillet over medium to medium-low
heat. Sweat the onions in the oil until very translucent and soft,
about 20 minutes. Stir often, and turn down heat if needed to
avoid crisping the onions. At the end of the sweating, add the butter and red wine to finish.

Make 3 very large, thin hamburger patties, using the ground sirloin.
Pan-broil them over medium-high heat, about 2 minutes on each
side, in the same skillet used to cook the onions. After cooking, cut
each patty into fours for each "slider." Top with Swiss cheese, and
add grape tomatoes on the side. Cover with mustard if desired.

Makes 4 servings.

Hints:
- Sweating onions means that you cook them slowly, with mini-
  mal browning. This brings out all the sweet flavor of the onions.
- If your kids don't like onions, leave them off their portion. And
  let them have slider buns.
- Great sides would be green beans and coleslaw.

Taco Salad

1 pound extra-lean ground sirloin
1 cup diced onions, frozen or fresh
1 cup red, yellow, and/or orange bell pepper strips, frozen or
    fresh
1 teaspoon chili powder
1 teaspoon paprika
½ teaspoon onion powder
½ teaspoon garlic powder
dash cayenne pepper, to taste
4 cups lettuce
1 cup grated carrots
3 tomatoes, cut into chunks
1 cucumber, diced
1½ cups sweet corn
4 ounces shredded Monterey Jack cheese

Heat a large nonstick skillet over medium-high heat. Add the
ground beef, onions, and peppers, cook 3 minutes, and turn down
the heat to medium. Stir occasionally while continuing to cook
until the meat is completely browned. Turn down the heat again
to medium-low and add the seasonings.

Plate the lettuce, and top with carrots, tomatoes, cucumber, and
sweet corn. Place the taco meat and then the cheese on top.

Makes 4 servings.

Hints: You can vary any of the seasonings according to your own
taste preferences.

For a vegetarian alternative, use soy-based crumbles, or canned,
drained black or kidney beans.

The World's Best Meatloaf

1 cup diced onions
½ cup diced carrots
½ cup diced celery
1 tablespoon butter or margarine
1 tablespoon olive oil
1 cup bread crumbs or oatmeal
2 pounds ground beef chuck
1 pound ground pork
6 ounces reduced-fat, sharp cheddar cheese
2 large eggs
½ cup beef bouillon
2 cloves pureed garlic
1 teaspoon salt
½ teaspoon pepper
2 teaspoons thyme
2 teaspoons paprika
1 teaspoon allspice
1 teaspoon oregano
3 bay leaves

Preheat the oven to 350°F.

In a nonstick skillet, sauté the onions, carrots, and celery in the oil and butter or margarine, about 5 minutes, until tender and translucent. Raise heat and sauté a few minutes longer, until lightly browned. Scrape into a large mixing bowl. Combine all the ingredients except the bay leaves in the bowl and mix together thoroughly with your clean hands. (You may want to remove your rings first.) Shape the mixture in the meatloaf loaf pan. Arrange the bay leaves on top.

Place the meatloaf pan on a baking sheet before putting it in the oven. (This helps prevent drips and spills.) Bake in the lower middle of the oven for about 1½ hours. The meatloaf is done when the juices run almost clear with a pale pink tinge. A meat thermometer should read 155°. Let cool for 30 minutes. If you have not used the double meatloaf pan, pour off any residual meat juices.

Makes about 10 servings.

Hints: We use a double meatloaf pan, which has slots in the inner pan, allowing the fats and juices to drop into the outer pan. It makes for a much leaner meatloaf.

Using the optional oatmeal instead of the bread crumbs will increase the fiber content.

Note: This recipe was adapted from Julia Child's *The Way to Cook*.

Mango-Berry Salsa with Grilled Pork Loin

1 tablespoon reduced-sodium soy sauce
3 cloves garlic, minced
¼ teaspoon black pepper
1½-to-2-pound boneless pork top loin roast (single loin)
1 mango, peeled and diced (about 1 cup)
¼ cup diced onion
2 tablespoons brown sugar or Splenda Brown Sugar
    Blend
1 finely diced small, fresh banana pepper
½ teaspoon lime zest
1 tablespoon lime juice
⅛ teaspoon salt
1 cup fresh raspberries or other berries

In a small bowl combine the soy sauce, garlic, and black pepper. Trim any excess fat from the meat. Use a sharp knife to cut (score) the outside of the top and bottom of the roast, making cuts about ¼-inch deep. Rub garlic mixture evenly onto all sides of meat. Insert a meat thermometer near the center of roast.

Preheat a grill with a cover to low-medium. Place the meat in a roasting pan on the grill rack. Cover and grill for about 1 hour or until a meat thermometer registers 155°F.

Remove the meat from the grill to a cutting board. Cover the meat with foil; let stand 15 minutes before carving. (The meat's temperature will rise 5°F during standing.)

Meanwhile, in a small bowl combine half of the chopped mango with the onion, brown sugar, banana pepper, lime zest, lime juice, and salt. Tear off a 24-by-18-inch piece of heavy foil. Fold in half to make a double thickness of foil that measures 18 by 12 inches. Spoon the mixture onto the center of the foil. Bring up two opposite edges of the foil. Fold the foil to enclose the mixture, leaving space for steam to build.

Place the mango packet on the rack of an uncovered grill for 10 minutes, or until heated through. Remove from heat. Transfer the grilled mango mixture to a medium bowl. Gently stir the remaining chopped mango and the raspberries into the grilled mango mixture. Serve with pork and, if desired, lime wedges.

Makes 6 servings.

Poultry

Naked Chicken Piccata
Super-Easy, Lip-Smacking-Good, Roasted Chicken and
    Winter Vegetables
Asian Chicken Lettuce Wraps
Southwestern Blackened Chicken Salad
Chicken Souvlaki
Poached Chicken Salad with Grapes and Walnuts
The Easiest Chicken Giardinara
Crispy Grilled Chicken

Chicken, Pan-Broiled, with Tomato and Broccoli Salad

Garden Splendor, Sautéed Chicken with Tomatoes over Haricots Verts

Blackened Chicken with Avocado-Papaya Salsa

Blackened Chicken and Berry Salad

Stand-up Chicken

Sesame Chicken Salad

Crispy Chicken Tenders

Turkey Roll-ups with Blueberry Salsa

Naked Chicken Piccata

It's called naked because there is no breading or capers. No breading to minimize refined starches, and no capers to keep sodium under control.

4 boneless, skinless chicken breasts
lemon-pepper seasoning mix
1 tablespoon olive oil
2 tablespoons lemon juice
½ teaspoon lemon zest
1 tablespoon butter or margarine
1 cup low-sodium chicken broth, preheated in a microwave

First, pound the chicken breasts with a wooden mallet until they are about ¼-inch thick. This will be easiest if you place them on sheets of plastic wrap and sprinkle water around the sheets so they don't stick so much. You could also use a rolling pin to thin and even out the breasts.

Sprinkle the breasts with the lemon-pepper seasoning mix. Heat the oil over medium-high heat. (If the oil is smoking, the cooking temperature is too high.) Add the chicken and cook about 4 minutes on each side, or until browned. Remove the chicken from the pan, and place on a plate with a cover (such as a pot lid or aluminum foil) to keep warm.

Add the lemon juice, zest, and hot chicken broth to the skillet, scraping the pan to loosen any browned bits. Continue to cook to thicken the sauce. Reduce the heat and add the butter or margarine. Return the chicken to the pan and cook about another 3 minutes, or until the internal temperature of the breasts is at least 165°F.

Makes 4 servings.

Hint: To make this dish even lower in sodium, use 1 cup of white wine instead of the chicken broth. You will still have great flavor.

Super-Easy, Lip-Smacking-Good, Roasted Chicken and Winter Vegetables

1 roasting chicken, 5–6 pounds
poultry seasonings
15 new red potatoes (very small)
12-ounce bag frozen crinkle cut carrots
12-ounce bag frozen Brussels sprouts
1 medium onion, cut into chunks
4 cloves garlic, minced or smashed
1 can low-sodium chicken broth
parsley, dried or finely chopped fresh
1 tablespoon olive oil

Preheat oven to 450°F.

Clean the chicken, removing all the giblets and the neck (if included). Pat dry. Sprinkle poultry seasonings over the inside and outside of the bird. Place the bird on the rack in a roaster. Place the potatoes, carrots, and Brussels sprouts on the bottom of the roaster. Place onion chunks around and inside the bird. Add minced garlic around the bottom of the pan and inside the bird. Sprinkle parsley over the bird and vegetables, then drizzle with olive oil.

Roast in the oven for 30 minutes, then reduce heat to 350°F. Roast for another 45 minutes, or until thermometer inserted deep into the breast reads 165°F. The bird should be a deep golden brown. If the liquid on the bottom dries out, add additional water to keep the vegetables from burning.

Makes 6 servings.

Hints: You can choose almost any type of vegetable, fresh or frozen, that you like. And cut-up sweet potatoes would be interesting instead of the red potatoes.

This recipe would also work well in a slow cooker.

Asian Chicken Lettuce Wraps

2 tablespoons low-sodium light soy sauce
1 tablespoon hoisin sauce (plum sauce)
2 tablespoons rice wine vinegar
½ teaspoon sugar or Splenda
3 tablespoons canola or peanut oil (no peanut oil if you have an allergy to peanuts)
2 cloves garlic, minced
2 teaspoons minced fresh ginger or 2 dashes of ground ginger
⅓ cup diced red onion
1 cup chopped button mushrooms
½ cup water chestnuts, diced
1 pound boneless, skinless chicken breasts, diced or cut in strips
8–10 inner leaves chilled iceberg lettuce
fresh cilantro leaves, coarsely chopped (optional)
¼ cup unsalted roasted cashews, coarsely chopped (skip if you have nut allergies)

Combine the soy sauce, hoisin sauce, vinegar, and sugar in a small bowl and mix together until the sugar dissolves.

Heat 1 tablespoon of the oil in a wok or skillet over medium-high to high heat. (If the oil smokes, turn down the heat. The smoke is hazardous to your lungs.) Mix the garlic and ginger into the oil, then add the onion, mushrooms, and water chestnuts. Stir-fry for 2 minutes, then remove from the wok.

Heat the remaining 2 tablespoons of oil in the wok. Add the chicken and brown for 1 minute, or until no longer pink. Add the cooked vegetable mixture back to the wok, decrease the heat, and stir in the sauce mixture. Stir for 1 minute, or until the sauce is heated and the chicken is cooked through.

Spoon the filling into each of the lettuce cups. Top each lettuce cup with cilantro and sprinkle with chopped cashews (if desired). Serve warm.

Makes about 4 servings.

Hint: Peanut oil works very well for high-temperature cooking since it is more resistant to smoking. Canola or safflower oil are also good.

Southwestern Blackened Chicken Salad

2 ripe medium tomatoes, peeled and diced
2 tablespoons finely diced red onion
2 tablespoons finely chopped fresh cilantro
dash of sugar (optional)
4 medium skinless, boneless chicken breasts (about 1 pound)
4 teaspoons ground black pepper
4 teaspoons paprika
¾ teaspoon dry mustard
¾ teaspoon ground red pepper
¼ teaspoon salt
shredded lettuce (about 4 cups, or per your preference)
1 cup sweet corn (except during Phase 1)
4 ounces shredded cheddar or Monterey Jack cheese
guacamole

Preheat oven to 350°F.

For your homemade Pico de Gallo: Combine the tomatoes, red onion, cilantro, and sugar. Mix well. Cover; chill for several hours or overnight.

Cut chicken breast halves into ¾-inch-wide strips. Combine the black pepper, paprika, dry mustard, red pepper, and salt in a plastic bag. Add chicken to the bag, shaking to coat. Arrange coated chicken in a single layer in a shallow baking pan, either sprayed with cooking spray, or lined with nonstick aluminum foil. Bake, uncovered, for 15–20 minutes, or until the chicken is tender and no longer pink. Using two forks, shred the chicken into pieces.

Arrange the lettuce on plates, sprinkle with corn (not in Phase 1), and top with shredded chicken. Spread Pico de Gallo, cheddar or Monterey Jack cheese, and guacamole on top of the chicken and lettuce. And who said healthy eating can't be super-tasty!

Makes 4 servings.

Hint: To peel tomatoes, make an X cut on the bottom of each tomato. Using a slotted ladle, slip into boiling water, until the skin softens and starts peel back from the X (30–45 seconds). Remove with the ladle, then plunge into ice water to stop the cooking. You will then be easily able to peel off the skin. If you are in a pinch and don't have any flavorful tomatoes, you could substitute whole canned tomatoes.

Chicken Souvlaki

3 lemons
2 tablespoons finely chopped fresh oregano leaves or 2 teaspoons dry oregano
½ teaspoon crushed red pepper flakes
¼ cup olive oil
4 cloves garlic, minced
coarse salt
16 chicken tenders (tenderloins), about 1½ pounds
ground black pepper
2 cups Greek-style yogurt
½ seedless cucumber, peeled and grated
½ teaspoon ground cumin

You will need about 16 skewers. If you are using bamboo ones, soak in water for about 30 minutes prior to grilling.

Preheat grill to medium-high heat.

To prepare the marinade, combine the zest and juice of 2 lemons, oregano, red pepper flakes, and olive oil in a dish. Paste the garlic by mashing it with a little coarse salt (such as Kosher salt or sea salt) then add ¾ of it to the marinade, reserving some for the dipping sauce. Add the chicken tenders to the marinade in a large ziplock bag and season with the pepper, shake in the marinade to coat, and let stand about 10 minutes.

Thread the tenders on the skewers and cook 7–8 minutes, turning once, until firm and juices run clear.

While the chicken cooks, combine the yogurt with the juice of the remaining lemon and the reserved garlic, grated cucumber, and cumin. Serve the dip to be used as desired as a dip or sauce for the chicken.

Makes about 4 servings.

Hint: Microplanes are the best and easiest graters for citrus peel. Zest first, then remove the juice. Don't skip the zest, because it adds such a clean, intense flavor.

Poached Chicken Salad with Grapes and Walnuts

5 cups water
1¾ cups low-sodium chicken broth
1½ pounds chicken tenders
⅓ cup plain nonfat yogurt
⅓ cup mayonnaise
1 tablespoon Dijon mustard
1 cup seedless grapes, cut in half, crosswise
1 cup coarsely chopped walnuts (3 ounces)
Salt and pepper to taste

Bring water and broth to a boil in a large saucepan, then add chicken and cook at a bare simmer, uncovered, stirring occasionally, until just cooked through, about 5 minutes. Drain and cool, then cut into 1-inch chunks.

Combine the yogurt, mayonnaise, and mustard. Stir the chicken and remaining ingredients into the dressing with salt and pepper to taste.

Makes 6 servings.

Hint: This is great served on lettuce, with sliced tomatoes.

The Easiest Chicken Giardinara

1 tablespoon olive oil
4 chicken breasts, boneless, skinless
12 ounces canned giardinara
1 clove garlic, minced

Recapping from the Naked Chicken Piccata recipe: First, pound the chicken breasts with a wooden mallet until they are about ¼-inch thick. This will be easiest if you place them on sheets of plastic wrap and sprinkle water around the sheets so they don't stick so much. You could also use a rolling pin to thin and even out the breasts.

Heat the oil over medium-high heat. (If the oil is smoking, the cooking temperature is too high.) Add the chicken and cook about 4 minutes on each side, or until browned. Remove the chicken from the pan and place on a plate with a cover (such as a pot lid or aluminum foil) to keep warm.

Into a skillet, add the giardinara and garlic. Sauté over medium heat for 2–3 minutes, or until hot. Add back the chicken and cover with the giardinara-garlic mixture. Simmer for another 2 minutes. Serve hot.

Makes 4 servings.

Warning: This dish is very spicy!

Crispy Grilled Chicken

4 chicken breasts, bone-in, with skin
Optional: garlic clove or salt-free seasoning mix

Heat the barbecue grill to medium heat. Create a boat out of aluminum foil for each of the chicken breasts. If desired, for extra flavor, rub the chicken with a peeled, cut garlic clove or sprinkle with salt-free seasoning mix. Place chicken, skin side down, in boats. Cook for 45 minutes, turning the chicken in the boats every 15 minutes.

You will get a lovely, golden brown color, and intense flavor from the caramelization of the chicken skin. And does it get any easier?

Makes 4 servings.

Hint: Use nonstick aluminum foil for the boats.

Chicken, Pan-Broiled, with Tomato and Broccoli Salad

1½ pounds boneless, skinless chicken breasts
4 cups broccoli florets
1½ pounds medium tomatoes
4 tablespoons olive or canola oil
½ teaspoon salt
1 teaspoon freshly ground pepper
½ teaspoon chili powder
¼ cup lemon juice

Place the chicken in a skillet and add enough water to cover; bring to a simmer over high heat. Cover, reduce heat, and simmer gently until the chicken is cooked through and is no longer pink in the middle, 10–12 minutes. Transfer to a cutting board. When cool enough to handle, shred with two forks into bite-sized pieces.

Microwave the broccoli about 5 minutes, or until tender. Allow to cool uncovered.

Cut the tomatoes in half lengthwise. Do not remove the seeds and pulp, since this is where most of the flavor is. In the skillet used for cooking the chicken, preheat 1 tablespoon of the olive oil and sauté the tomatoes over medium-high heat, starting with the cut side down. Allow to brown, and soften. Turn and brown on the other side. Remove to a plate to cool.

Heat the remaining 3 tablespoons of oil in the pan over medium heat. Stir in the salt, pepper, and chili powder and cook, stirring constantly, until fragrant, about 45 seconds. Slowly pour in the lemon juice (watch out for splatters), then remove the pan from the heat. Stir to scrape up any browned bits.

Coarsely chop the pan-broiled tomatoes and combine them in a large bowl with the shredded chicken, broccoli, and pan dressing; toss to coat.

Makes 4 servings.

Garden Splendor, Sautéed Chicken with Tomatoes over Haricots Verts

2 tablespoons olive or canola oil

8 thin-cut boneless, skinless chicken breasts

3 cups haricots verts (very thin whole green beans)

2 cups cherry or grape tomatoes, cut in halves

1–2 cloves garlic, minced or crushed through a garlic press, or ½ teaspoon minced garlic (optional)

1 cup frozen diced onions

1 tablespoon minced fresh basil (or 1 teaspoon dried basil)

1 tablespoon minced fresh oregano (or about 1 teaspoon dried oregano, or to taste)

1 tablespoon minced fresh Italian parsley (or 1 teaspoon dried parsley flakes)

4 ounces chicken broth, low-sodium, or white wine

Preheat the oven (or a toaster oven) to 250°F.

This recipe idea originally came from foods we had on hand, including our garden bounty. This was a great way to utilize our excess Super Sweet 100 mini cherry tomatoes from the garden. It makes a lovely meal, with a sauce pulled together from your garden or from the market.

Preheat the oil in a nonstick skillet over medium-high heat. Brown the chicken, sautéing in the oil. (You may be able to do only 2–4 breasts at a time, depending on the size of your skillet.) Turn the heat down to medium after 1 minute of cooking. Turn the chicken after 2–3 minutes and continue to cook another 2 minutes. Remove and place on an oven-safe dish. Cover with aluminum foil or a pot lid, and keep warm in the oven or toaster oven. There will be a slight continuation of the cooking process, so don't overcook the chicken during the browning process. Repeat this process until you have cooked all the chicken.

Immediately start cooking the green beans in a microwave, for about 5 minutes.

Then add the cut-up mini cherry tomatoes, garlic, and frozen diced onions to the skillet, and sauté on medium-low heat. Season with basil, oregano, and Italian parsley. Add the chicken broth (or white wine to eliminate the sodium) and continue to cook down the liquid to thicken slightly. Add all the chicken back into the skillet and spoon the sauce over it.

Place the chicken on top of the beans, and top with the sauce. This is an easy way to also season the beans, without any extra effort.

Makes 4 servings.

Hints: We like to use homegrown Super Sweet 100 mini cherry tomatoes. These tomato vines are prodigious, so we always have lots of very flavorful tomatoes during the summer and fall.

The thin-cut chicken breasts are much easier to cook because they have a uniform thickness. You could use any skinless, boneless chicken breasts, but they may take a little longer to cook, or pound them thin as if you were making Naked Chicken Piccata.

You could mince all the herbs (except the garlic) at one time to reduce your prep time.

Blackened Chicken with Avocado-Papaya Salsa

4 skinless, boneless chicken breasts
2 teaspoons blackened steak seasoning
3 tablespoons olive oil
2 tablespoons rice wine vinegar
¼ teaspoon ground cumin
dash ground black pepper
1 avocado, halved, seeded, peeled, and medium chopped
⅔ cup fresh or refrigerated papaya (without added sugar),
    diced
⅓ cup diced red bell pepper
¼ cup chopped fresh cilantro (optional)

Preheat the oven to 375°F.

Lightly sprinkle both sides of each chicken breast half with blackened steak seasoning. In a large oven-safe skillet (no plastic handle), heat 1 tablespoon of the oil over medium heat. Add the chicken; cook until browned, turning once. Cook about 15 minutes, or until the chicken is no longer pink (165°F).

For the salsa: In a large bowl, whisk together the rice vinegar, the remaining 2 tablespoons of oil, the cumin, and the black pepper. Stir in the avocado, papaya, red bell pepper, and chopped cilantro. Serve the chicken topped with the salsa.

Makes 4 servings.

Blackened Chicken and Berry Salad

4 chicken breasts, boneless, skinless
blackening spice mixture
1 tablespoon olive or canola oil
2–3 cups lettuce mix (per your preferences)
2 medium tomatoes, cut into wedges, or substitute grape
    tomatoes

½ cup shredded red cabbage
½ cup shredded carrots
1 cup sliced strawberries
1 cup red raspberries
1 cup blueberries
French vinaigrette dressing

Rinse the chicken breasts and blot dry with a paper towel. Put the spice mixture on a plate and dredge the breasts through the mixture. Preheat the oil in a skillet over medium-high heat. Sear both sides of the chicken, cooking 2–3 minutes per side. Then reduce the heat until the chicken is fully cooked. (Hint: Alternately, the chicken could be cooked on a grill.) Let cool a few minutes, then slice into 1-inch strips, crosswise.

Arrange your lettuce on plates and cover with tomatoes, red cabbage, and shredded carrots. Then place the chicken strips on each salad and top with a variety of the berries. Dress with the vinaigrette.

Makes 4 servings.

Stand-up Chicken

Special equipment is needed for this recipe. We use an upright roasting stand, also known as a vertical chicken roaster. Some people use a half-full beer can as a roaster. They claim that the beer steams the inside while roasting, leaving a moister chicken.

1 roasting chicken
poultry seasonings
paprika
½ cup liquid of your choice (water, broth, wine, etc.)

Preheat the oven to 425°F.

Take out the top rack of your oven and ensure that the bottom rack is on its lowest level. (Since the chicken will be vertical, you need maximum headroom in the oven.) Rinse the chicken and pat dry. Sprinkle with seasonings, inside and out. Put the chicken on the vertical roaster, and then set in a pan. (We often use a glass pie pan. It fits nicely.) Put about ½ cup of liquid in the bottom of the pan. You could use water, beer, wine, chicken broth, etc. Keep watching during cooking to ensure that you still have liquid in the pan. Add more as needed. Place in the oven and cook for about 70 minutes, or until a meat thermometer registers 165°F inside the breast. The chicken should be a deep golden brown.

Makes 4–6 servings.

Hint: This is a super-easy dish and gives you time to relax or exercise while the chicken cooks.

Sesame Chicken Salad

3 tablespoons canola oil
3 tablespoons rice wine vinegar
1 tablespoon minced fresh ginger
black pepper to taste
½ cup Dijon mustard
⅓ cup maple syrup
1½ pounds chicken tenders
½ cup sesame seeds
1 bag mixed greens
½ seedless cucumber, unpeeled, sliced thinly into rounds
2 large tomatoes, cut into 8 wedges

To make the dressing, mix 2 tablespoons of the canola oil, the rice vinegar, and the ginger in bowl. Season with pepper to taste.

Mix the mustard and syrup in a bowl, add the chicken, and marinate 1 hour. Then spread the sesame seeds on a plate. As you remove the chicken from the marinade, shake off any excess. Coat the chicken on both sides with the sesame seeds. Discard the marinade; do not reuse! Sprinkle the chicken with pepper. Heat 1 tablespoon of the oil in a large nonstick skillet over medium-high heat. Working in batches, add the chicken to the skillet and sauté until just cooked through, about 2 minutes per side. Add more oil to the skillet if needed. Transfer the chicken to a plate.

Mix the greens, cucumber, and tomatoes in a large bowl. Toss to coat with dressing. Place the salad on each of the plates, top with the chicken, and serve.

Makes 4 servings.

Crispy Chicken Tenders

  salt-free seasoning mix
  1½ pounds chicken tenders
  1 tablespoon olive oil

Place a layer of seasoning mix on a plate, then dredge the tenders through the mix. Add oil to a skillet over medium-high heat. Cook the tenders 2–3 minutes on each side, or until golden brown.

Serving ideas: Have the tenders on a salad with lots of veggies. Serve them as a main course, with side vegetables and coleslaw. Shred, top with salsa and lettuce, and roll up in soft corn tortillas for an interesting chicken taco.

Makes 4–5 servings.

Hint: Make an extra batch at the same time, to freeze for later use.

We like Costco's Kirkland Organic Salt-Free Seasonings. And there are many other good salt-free mixes.

Turkey Roll-ups with Blueberry Salsa

2 cups coarsely chopped fresh blueberries
1 cup whole fresh blueberries
¼ cup lemon juice
3 tablespoons chopped fresh cilantro (optional)
2 jalapeños, seeded and minced
⅓ cup diced red bell pepper
¼ cup finely diced onion
8 small (6-inch) whole wheat or corn tortillas (or lettuce leaves)
1 pound turkey, thinly sliced

Stir together the chopped and the whole blueberries, lemon juice, cilantro, jalapeños, bell pepper, and onion in a large bowl. Cover and chill until ready to serve.

Create each roll-up with a tortilla (or lettuce leaf), 2 ounces of turkey, and a strip of the blueberry salsa down the center. Then roll up and enjoy!

Makes 8 roll-ups, or 3–4 servings.

Hint: If you make extra salsa, you can use it for other meals.

Fish and Seafood

Alaska Walnut-Crusted Salmon with Raspberry Coulis
Acapulco Tuna Salad
Fish Tacos
Baked Salmon with Honey
Baked Halibut with Sherry
Tilapia with Salsa

Alaska Walnut-Crusted Salmon
with Raspberry Coulis

1–1½ pounds salmon filet, skin removed
1 tablespoon mayonnaise
1 cup finely chopped walnuts
2 cups raspberries, fresh or frozen
¼ cup sugar
1 tablespoon lemon juice
1 teaspoon lemon zest

Preheat the oven to 350°F.

Place the salmon filet, presentation side up, on a baking sheet covered in nonstick aluminum foil or parchment paper. Cover very thinly with the mayonnaise. Then gently press the walnuts onto the layer of mayonnaise. Bake for 15–20 minutes, or until the salmon flakes with a fork.

Prepare the coulis by heating the raspberries with the sugar in a medium saucepan over medium-high heat. Lower the heat and simmer, stirring occasionally, until the mixture starts to thicken, about 15 minutes. Then press through a fine-mesh strainer (or a hand food mill), using a spatula to press out as much liquid as possible. Discard the seeds and skins. Stir in the lemon juice and zest.

Cut the salmon into 4 portions, plate, and top each serving with the raspberry coulis.

Makes 4 servings.

Hint: You can prepare the coulis earlier, and refrigerate 1–2 days, if needed.

Acapulco Tuna Salad

2 6-ounces cans tuna, very low sodium
2 tablespoons low-fat mayonnaise or regular mayonnaise made
 with olive oil
1 medium tomato, diced
½ small sweet onion, diced very finely
1 jalapeño, diced, seeds and spines removed
1 tablespoon lime juice

Drain the water from the tuna and mix all the ingredients in a medium bowl.

Makes 4 servings.

Fish Tacos

2 pounds tilapia
lemon-pepper seasoning mix
1 tablespoon olive or canola oil, or grill-safe cooking spray if
 cooking on a grill
8 whole wheat or corn tortillas, small (6-inch)
1 pat butter
lime wedges
shredded red cabbage

You have choices on how to cook the fish. You can either pan sauté or grill it. First, sprinkle with the lemon-pepper seasoning mix.

To pan sauté: Add the oil to a nonstick skillet preheated over medium to medium-high heat. Before adding the fish, be sure that it is dry, to avoid hot oil spatters. Sauté about 4 minutes per side or until the fish flakes. During last minute add a small pat of butter to finish the flavor.

To grill: Spray the grill with a cooking spray that is meant for the grill. Over medium-high heat, cook the fish about 4 minutes per side.

Serve hot, drizzle with the lime juice from wedges, and top with the red cabbage. The Mango-Melon Salsa* is also great to serve on the fish tacos, as are avocado slices.

Hint: If you are grilling the fish, use a fish-grilling pan, which has small holes all over and helps prevent the fish from flaking and getting stuck to the grill.

Makes 4 servings.

Baked Salmon with Honey

½ cup honey
3 tablespoons melted butter or margarine
3 tablespoons soy sauce, reduced-sodium
3 tablespoons fresh lemon juice
1 tablespoon lemon zest
2 tablespoons white wine
2 pounds salmon filet

Mix all the ingredients except the salmon in a 9-by-13-inch baking pan. Then place the salmon in the pan, cover, and marinate for 30 minutes to 6 hours in the refrigerator.

Preheat the oven to 400°F. Bake for 10–15 minutes, or until easily flaked with a fork. Baste a few times while baking. Serve immediately.

Makes 6 servings.

Baked Halibut with Sherry

vegetable oil spray
1 tablespoon olive oil
1 medium Bermuda onion, thinly sliced
2 cloves garlic, minced
3 tablespoons sherry wine (can substitute other wine if not available)
1½ pounds halibut filets
1 15.5-ounce can vegetable stock or low-sodium chicken stock
fresh-ground pepper
1 teaspoon lemon zest

Preheat the oven to 425°F.

Spray a baking dish with vegetable oil spray. Heat the oil and onion in a sauté pan over medium heat. Taking care to avoid burning the onions, cook about 10 minutes, until golden brown. Lower the heat to medium-low and add the minced garlic and sherry; cook another 3 minutes.

Place the halibut in a single layer in a baking pan, add stock, sprinkle with the lemon zest, and bake for 10–15 minutes, or until the fish easily flakes with a fork. Serve each filet topped with sherry-onion sauce.

Makes 4 servings.

Tilapia with Salsa

2 diced medium tomatoes (in winter, you can use no-added-salt diced tomatoes)
½ medium Vidalia onion, diced
1 medium jalapeño, veins and seeds removed, minced
1 tablespoon chopped cilantro
1 teaspoon sugar
1 tablespoon red vinegar
4 tilapia filets

To make the salsa, combine all the ingredients except the tilapia. The fish can be cooked either on the grill or in a sauté pan. To grill, use a fish grill pan and cover with vegetable oil spray, to prevent excessive sticking. Top with salsa and cook about 3 minutes. Then flip the fish, top again with salsa, and cook for another 3 minutes, or until the fish is cooked through and flakes easily with a fork.

Makes 4 servings.

Hint: If you are pressed for time, a commercial salsa can be used. This is a great way to add flavor to a very mild-tasting fish.

Vegetarian

The Frittata That Makes a Meal
Creamy Cauliflower Mashed Potatoes
Mashed Sweet Potatoes with Maple and Orange
Green Beans with Toasted Almond Slivers
Glazed Carrots
Roasted Brussels Sprouts with Balsamic Dressing
Roasted Broccoli, Cauliflower, and Carrots
Romaine and Blood Orange Salad
Green Beans and Peppers
Zucchini Lasagna
Mango-Melon Salsa

The Frittata That Makes a Meal

6 whole large eggs (or equivalent egg substitutes)
1 teaspoon dry basil (or 1 tablespoon diced fresh basil)

2 tablespoons canola or olive oil
1 cup sliced bell peppers
¼ cup sliced onion
1 cup frozen extra-sweet corn
1 cup grape or cherry tomatoes, halved
4 ounces shredded Colby-Jack cheese or other cheese blend

Lightly stir the eggs. Add the basil.

Pour the oil into a nonstick frying pan with a metal handle, over medium heat. When the oil is hot, add the pepper strips, onion, and corn. (You can substitute a frozen mixture of pepper strips and onions, instead of fresh, if desired.) Sauté for 3 minutes, with frequent stirring. Then add the tomatoes and continue to stir. Cook an additional 5 minutes, or until the onions are translucent.

Pour the egg-basil mixture over the vegetables. Use a spatula to lift the edges or separate slightly in the interior, and allow the eggs to fall to the bottom of mixture as the frittata cooks. When egg mixture is thickened all the way through, top with cheese. Then brown under a broiler for 2–3 minutes.

Makes 6 servings.

Hint: Be sure to use a pan with a metal handle; plastic will melt under the broiler. We used an All-Clad pan.

Creamy Cauliflower Mashed Potatoes

1 medium head cauliflower (or frozen florets), to make about 8 cups
4 cloves garlic, peeled (optional)
⅓ cup skim milk, buttermilk, or nonfat sour cream (not containing titanium dioxide)
1 pat soft butter or margarine, about 1 teaspoon

½ teaspoon salt
pepper to taste

Chop the cauliflower into florets. Place them in boiling water in a saucepan along with the garlic, if desired, and cook about 6 minutes, or until soft.

Drain off the liquid and put the florets in a blender, food processor, or medium bowl. Add about half of the skim milk (or buttermilk, or nonfat sour cream) and the butter or margarine. Puree mechanically or by hand until mostly creamy but with some slight lumps for texture. Add the extra liquid as needed during the blending. Add salt and pepper to taste.

Makes 4 servings.

Hint: You can also use a microwave. Cook 5 minutes on high, or until soft. Stir halfway through the cooking cycle.

Mashed Sweet Potatoes with Maple and Orange

4–5 large sweet potatoes or yams
½ cup heated milk
1 ounce butter or margarine
¼ cup maple syrup
⅓ cup orange juice
1 tablespoon orange zest

Preheat the oven to 400°F.

Place the sweet potatoes on a baking sheet covered with nonstick aluminum foil, and bake until well softened, about 60 minutes. (Hint: My clue that they are done is when I start to see sugar seeping out of the potatoes.)

Let cool a few minutes, then cut in half, lengthwise. Scoop out the interiors or peel away the exteriors and place in a large bowl.

Start to mash the potatoes, then add ¼ cup of the heated milk, the butter or margarine, syrup, orange juice, and zest. Continue to mash until you have your desired consistency. Add the rest of the milk if needed.

Makes about 8 servings.

Green Beans with Toasted Almond Slivers

½ cup almond slivers
1 bag frozen haricots verts (very thin, whole French green beans)
1 tablespoon olive oil
1 thin pat of butter

Preheat a toaster oven (or a regular oven) to 350°F.

Toast the almond slivers on a toaster pan or baking sheet about 10 minutes, or until you smell the almond fragrance.

Either microwave or quickly boil the green beans until slightly softened. Drain (if needed), drizzle with olive oil, and top with the pat of butter. Sprinkle the almond slivers over the top.

Makes 4 servings.

Glazed Carrots

¼ cup margarine
1 tablespoon brown sugar
1 tablespoon honey
¼ teaspoon nutmeg
½ teaspoon cinnamon
6–7 medium carrots, peeled, cut into 1-inch diagonally sliced sections

fresh minced parsley and/or chives

In a medium skillet, melt the margarine over medium heat, taking care to avoid burning. Add the brown sugar, honey, nutmeg, and cinnamon; mix together. Add the carrots. Cover; cook on medium-low to medium heat about 15 minutes, stirring occasionally. If you prefer softer carrots, continue cooking until your texture preference is reached. Serve hot, topped with the parsley or chives.

Makes 4 servings.

Roasted Brussels Sprouts with Balsamic Dressing

3 tablespoons balsamic vinegar
1 teaspoon onion powder
½ teaspoon ground black pepper
3 tablespoons olive oil
1 bag frozen Brussels sprouts, or 2–3 cups fresh

Preheat the oven to 375°F.

Whisk the vinegar, onion powder, and pepper in a small bowl. Slowly add the olive oil and whisk well after each addition.

Place the Brussels sprouts in a single layer on a baking sheet covered with nonstick aluminum foil. Drizzle the dressing over the sprouts, coating well. Bake for 25 minutes, turning once about midway through. The sprouts are done when they are moderately soft and are mildly browned in spots.

Makes 4 servings.

Hint: Instead of the onion powder, you could add diced or sliced onions to the Brussels sprouts and allow them to roast and add more intense flavor.

Roasted Broccoli, Cauliflower, and Carrots

2 medium stalks broccoli, cut into florets
1 small head cauliflower, cut into florets
4 large carrots, sliced into about 1-inch chunks
cooking spray, preferably olive oil
paprika
3 cloves garlic, thinly sliced

Preheat the oven to 425°F.

Line a baking sheet with nonstick aluminum foil. In a single layer, place the broccoli, cauliflower, and carrots. Spray with the cooking spray, then sprinkle with the paprika and garlic slices. Bake 25–30 minutes.

Makes 4–5 servings.

Hint: You could use a bag of frozen mixed cauliflower, broccoli, and carrots if you are pressed for time.

Romaine and Blood Orange Salad

4 cups sliced romaine lettuce hearts
3 blood oranges, peeled and sliced
½ cup pomegranate seeds
2 tablespoons lemon juice
1 tablespoon extra virgin olive oil
1 tablespoon honey
1½ teaspoons vanilla
dash salt
ground black pepper to taste
dash cinnamon
3 tablespoons slivered almonds (or crispy rice noodles if you have a nut allergy)

Top the lettuce with the blood orange slices and pomegranate seeds. Mix the rest of the ingredients except the almonds (or noodles). Dress the salad with the dressing and top with the almonds or noodles.

Makes 4 servings.

Adapted from Paula Wolfert's *The Food of Morocco.*

Green Beans and Peppers

1 tablespoon olive oil
8 ounces (by weight) whole green beans
1 each red, yellow, and orange bell peppers cut into strips
1 clove garlic, minced

Preheat the oil in a skillet over medium-high heat. Add the beans and peppers. Sauté, stirring occasionally, until soft. Add the minced garlic as you are getting close to your desired degree of softness or firmness, that is, nearer to the end of cooking. You will want to continue cooking about 3 minutes after adding the garlic.

Makes 4 servings.

Zucchini Lasagna

1 tablespoon olive oil
2 large zucchinis, sliced about ¼-inch thick
4 large tomatoes, sliced about ¼-inch thick
2 medium onions, sliced very thin
1 sprig fresh basil, 6–8 leaves, chopped or thinly sliced
Italian seasonings
ground black pepper
8 ounces shredded 2% mozzarella

Preheat the oven to 400°F.

In a 2½-quart oval bakeware dish (such as Corningware), pour the olive oil (or spray with olive oil cooking spray). Cover the bottom of the dish with sliced zucchini. Then, spread a layer of tomatoes and a layer of onions. Top with half of the sliced basil, Italian seasonings (or other herbs from your garden), and ground pepper. Then add a layer of about half the shredded cheese. Repeat (except for the olive oil).

Bake about 30 minutes. Let cool for 5 minutes before serving.

Makes 6 servings.

Hint: This recipe is especially great for using up end-of-summer veggies. An easy way to slice the basil is to roll up several leaves (stem edges inside), and then make thin slices. You end up with very thin strips, called a *chiffonade*.

Note: This recipe is adapted from Liz Manaster's *From A to Zucchini*.

Mango-Melon Salsa

   1 very ripe mango, diced
   ¼–½ cantaloupe, diced
   ¼ honeydew melon, diced
   ¼ pineapple, diced
   1 red pepper, diced
   1–2 jalapeño peppers, diced
   ¼ cup rice wine vinegar
   1 tablespoon brown sugar or Splenda Brown Sugar Blend
   1 teaspoon cilantro, finely chopped (optional)

Mix together in a medium bowl all of the fruit and peppers. In a separate small bowl, mix the vinegar, sugar, and cilantro. Then pour the vinegar mix over the fruit mixture. Toss, cover, and refrigerate for 1 hour.

Makes 8 servings.

Hint: Don't want to buy a lot of excess fruit? I buy packaged slices of the melons and pineapple. That way, I can also see and smell whether the fruit is really good. And it reduces the amount of cutting that you have to do, as well as reducing any waste.

APPENDIX A

Need Gluten-Free? Dairy-Free? Making DASH Work for You

It seems as though more and more people are developing food allergies or some degree of food intolerance. Fortunately, meal plans that are based on real foods or whole foods, such as the DASH diet, make it much easier to avoid allergens.

The most common food allergens are wheat (gluten), peanuts and tree nuts, dairy (cow's milk), fish and shellfish, soy, and eggs. Unfortunately, dairy and nuts are part of the key foods for the DASH Diet Weight Loss Solution. So we will need to find ways around the allergens for those of you who have sensitivities.

And we do recognize that there are a range of intolerances from severe, life-threatening allergies that trigger anaphylactic shock, to mild insensitivities that might cause sniffling, puffiness, or bloating when you consume certain foods.

Dairy

With dairy sensitivities, there are two possible triggers. Some people have a true allergy to cow's milk and its derivatives. Others may have lactose intolerance, which prevents them from consuming many dairy foods.

With a true allergy to cow's milk, the individual will want to avoid dairy foods, with possible exceptions for goat's milk products and other non-cow-sourced dairy foods. Some people will not be able to consume any dairy products, no matter what the source. Please follow your doctor's or dietitian's advice regarding dairy.

If you have lactose intolerance, you should be able to consume yogurt and cheese with no or minimal problems. In the production of yogurt, lactose is turned into lactic acid by the beneficial bacteria. And when cheese is processed, most of the lactose is removed when the curds and whey are separated (thank you, Miss Muffet). The curds are the solids used for making the cheese, and the lactose goes with the watery whey. Many people find that they can consume all dairy foods if they add Lactaid drops to their milk or use Lactaid milk. Others might be able to use acidophilus milk without having any symptoms.

Nondairy substitutes are fine; you just need to be sure that they have similar calcium and vitamin D levels as the dairy foods they replace. Also, you will want to avoid those products that are highly sweetened.

True Allergies

Most people who have true food allergies know how to work around these problems. Unfortunately, nuts are a common food allergen, although they are a great DASH diet food. If you can have avocados, they would be a great substitute, with similar nutrients as nuts. Otherwise, just forget about this food group and get your healthy fats from olive oil and/or fatty fish. You may need to have a few extra servings of fruits and veggies to be sure you are getting enough potassium.

If you have gluten sensitivity or true celiac disease, the DASH diet makes it very easy to accommodate your eating style. Since most foods in the diet are very close to their natural state, you will have fewer possible gluten-containing additives to be concerned about. Further, there are no grains in Phase One, and lower levels of pastries or baked goods in the complete plan than would be in the typical American diet. Of course, in Phase Two, any of the gluten-free grains that you enjoy can be used as wheat substitutes. Today, there are so many gluten-free foods that people find it very easy to adapt for the DASH plan.

Other types of food allergies, such as eggs, seafood, or beans, can be accommodated by making substitutions with foods having similar nutrients. If you have more complicated allergies or other food digestive issues, you may want to consult with a dietitian to adapt the DASH diet for your personal needs.

You Have Reached Your Goal—How to Maintain Your Weight

Congratulations! Your commitment to reaching your goal has paid off, and you are at your target for a healthy weight. You have learned to eat in a style that is much lighter and makes you feel great. You are exercising or doing some kind of physical activity on a regular basis. You look and feel years younger.

And of course, you want to maintain this feeling. The DASH Diet Weight Loss Solution will continue to be your model for healthy eating and activity. You just can expand your repertoire to occasionally include more of the starchy foods, such as the grains (mostly whole grains, of course) and starchy vegetables. However, you will still want to keep these to a minimum. Most of us are not physically active enough or young enough to burn off too much starch or extra sugar.

Once or twice a week, you can splurge a little bit, and add some potatoes, or maybe a wonderful dessert. As long as you are still following the plan relatively closely, your weight will stay stable. At first you will want to keep checking your weight relatively frequently. If it starts to creep up again, you are overdoing the starch or sugar, and you will want to follow Phase Two again for a week or so.

While it might seem fun to go back to your old way of eating, none of us can do this without regaining the weight. For most of us, our days are relatively sedentary, and we can't burn off a higher-calorie diet. Just remember how good you feel on this lighter eating plan.

If you would like additional meal plans to help with maintaining your weight, *The DASH Diet Action Plan* is a great guide, which has helped thousands of people.

Overview of Weight Maintenance Diet Patterns

The following table will help you understand the daily food group patterns for maintaining your weight with the DASH Diet Weight Loss Solution.

Food Group Servings Per Day for Weight Maintenance			
	Smaller appetite	*Moderate appetite*	*Larger appetite*
Nonstarchy vegetables	Unlimited		
Dairy	2–3	2–3	3–4
Nuts, beans, seeds	1–2	1–3	2–4
Lean meat, fish, poultry, eggs	5–6 ounces	6–8 ounces	8–11 ounces
Fats	1–2	2–3	3–4
Whole grains	2–3	2–3	3–4
Fruit	3–4	3–5	3–5
Refined grains, sweets	1–2, or less	2–3, or less	3–4, or less

U.S. to Metric Conversions

U.S. to Metric Conversions, Height

Inches	Centimeters	Inches	Centimeters	Inches	Centimeters
58	147	67	170	76	193
59	150	68	173	77	196
60	152	69	175	78	198
61	155	70	178	79	201
62	157	71	180	80	203
63	160	72	183	81	206
64	163	73	185	82	208
65	165	74	188		
66	168	75	191		

U.S. to Metric Conversions, Weight

Pounds	Kilograms
½ (8 ounces)	0.23
1 (16 ounces)	0.45
1 ½	0.68
2	0.91
2 ½	1.13
3	1.36

U.S., Imperial, and Metric Conversions, Weight

Pounds	Stones	Kilograms	Pounds	Stones	Kilograms
95	6.8	43.1	195	13.9	88.5
100	7.1	45.4	200	14.3	90.7
105	7.5	47.6	205	14.6	93.0
110	7.9	49.9	210	15.0	95.3
115	8.2	52.2	215	15.4	97.5
120	8.6	54.4	220	15.7	99.8
125	8.9	56.7	225	16.1	102.1
130	9.3	59.0	230	16.4	104.3
135	9.6	61.2	235	16.8	106.6
140	10.0	63.5	240	17.1	108.9
145	10.4	65.8	245	17.5	111.1
150	10.7	68.0	250	17.9	113.4
155	11.1	70.3	255	18.2	115.7
160	11.4	72.6	260	18.6	117.9
165	11.8	74.8	265	18.9	120.2
170	12.1	77.1	270	19.3	122.5
175	12.5	79.4	275	19.6	124.7
180	12.9	81.6	280	20.0	127.0
185	13.2	83.9	285	20.4	129.3
190	13.6	86.2	290	20.7	131.5

Pounds	Stones	Kilograms	Pounds	Stones	Kilograms
295	21.1	133.8	325	23.2	147.4
300	21.4	136.1	330	23.6	149.7
305	21.8	138.3	335	23.9	152.0
310	22.1	140.6	340	24.3	154.2
315	22.5	142.9	345	24.6	156.5
320	22.9	145.1	350	25.0	158.8

U.S. to Metric Conversions, Temperature

Degrees Fahrenheit	Degrees Celsius
300	149
325	163
350	177
375	191
400	204
425	218
450	232
475	246

U.S. to Metric Conversions, Volume (Dry and Liquid)

Teaspoons	Milliliters
1/4	1
1/2	2
1	5
3 (1 tablespoon)	15
6 (2 tablespoons)	30

U.S. to Metric Conversions, Volume (Liquid)

Fluid Ounces	Milliliters
1	30
2	60
3	90
4	120
5	150
6	180
7	210
8	240

The following information is provided as a point of reference:

U.S. Conversions, Volume

3 teaspoons = 1 tablespoon

2 tablespoons = 1 fluid ounce

8 fluid ounces = 1 cup

2 cups = 1 pint

2 pints = 1 quart

Imperial Conversions, Volume

10 fluid ounces = 1 cup

20 fluid ounces = 1 pint

40 fluid ounces = 1 quart

Note: Since this book does not contain any baking recipes (such as pastries, breads, cakes), precision is not important with the quantities. Typically in U.S. recipes, volumes, rather than weights, are used for most ingredients.

Additional DASH-Friendly Recipes

Beef, Pork, and Chicken

    https://www.beefitswhatsfordinner.com
    https://www.yummly.com/page/pork
    https://www.chickenroost.com

Seafood

    https://www.seafoodnutrition.org

Dairy

    https://www.nationaldairycouncil.org/farm-to-table
      #RecipesAnchor

Fruits and Vegetables

    https://fruitsandveggies.org/recipes

Plant-Based Protein

    https://www.almonds.com/consumers/recipe-center

https://www.Michiganbeans.org
https://pulses.org/nap/pulse-recipes
https://walnuts.org/recipes
https://www.soyconnection.com/recipes
http://www.soyfoods.com/category/recipes

Be sure to check my web page for more websites and updates on the above sites (since they often change their page names): http://dashdiet.org/dash_diet_recipe_links.

ACKNOWLEDGMENTS

I am so thrilled to be able to bring you this book. Many people have been supportive of this effort. First, my patients, in my private practice and at the Navy Hospital, inspired me to combine the benefits of the DASH diet with a more aggressive weight loss plan, especially targeted for people who need a lower carb diet plan.

My agent, Laurie Bernstein, was a powerhouse, championing the benefits of DASH and how powerful it could be when communicated in a way that was accessible to consumers and could fit into a real life. I was so lucky to become her client and to always have her strong support for spreading the word about the DASH diet and my books.

My editor, Diana Baroni, brought much enthusiasm to the project, both for the current books and the upcoming DASH books. I am very grateful for her providing the opportunity to share DASH with a world-wide market.

And of course, my husband, Richard, has been a rock, supporting all my work on the book, ready to try any of my new recipes, and never complaining when our "fun time" got interrupted by more work on the books. I have been so fortunate to have such a supportive, understanding, and loving husband. And, no one could hope for a husband who was more proud and eager to tell everyone about my works.

INDEX

ABOUT THE AUTHOR

Marla Heller, MS, RD, is a registered dietitian and holds a master of science in human nutrition and dietetics from the University of Illinois at Chicago (UIC), where she also completed doctoral course work in public health, with an emphasis in behavior sciences and health promotion. She is experienced in a wide variety of nutrition counseling specialties and has taught thousands of people how to adopt the DASH diet. She has been an adjunct clinical instructor in the Department of Human Nutrition and Dietetics at UIC, teaching courses on food science and nutrition counseling. At the University of Illinois Medical Center, she was a dietitian working in the Cardiac Step-Down Unit, the Cardiac Intensive Care Unit, and the Heart-Lung Transplant Unit. She was a civilian dietitian with the U.S. Navy and most recently worked for the U.S. Department of Health and Human Services, including the Healthy Weight Collaborative.

In addition to writing the *New York Times* bestseller *The DASH Diet Action Plan*, Marla contributed the four-week menu plan for *Win the Weight Game* by Sarah, the Duchess of York. She has been a featured nutrition expert for many national print, television, radio, Internet, and social media platforms.

She is a spokesperson for the Greater Midwest Affiliate of the American Heart Association and a past president of the Illinois Dietetic Association, from which she received their prestigious Emerging Leader Award.

Marla lives with her husband, Richard, and enjoys cooking, gardening, and finding exciting new restaurants.